# Yoga
## for Beauty
## and Health

by Eugene S. Rawls
and Eve Diskin

WARNER BOOKS

A Warner Communications Company

# DEDICATION

This book is fondly dedicated to women everywhere who are determined not to sit back and accept the loss of that wonderfully ageless beauty and vitality which can be easily theirs through Yoga.

# A MEDICAL DOCTOR'S FOREWORD

Through wise self-appraisal we can discover those areas in our complex natures which are weaker than others and which must be strengthened if we are to perform well in living up to life's challenges. This applies to our physical as well as our mental and moral make-up.

An obvious weakness that is becoming more general every day is the deterioration of our physical fitness, appearance and health. It is already axiomatic that too many of us "ride instead of walk" for reasonably short distances. People no longer ride horses, walk miles to work, play vigorously, climb, jump, run or bend as part of their everyday life. We are losing more and more of the necessary hardiness, and the positive qualities of body, mind and spirit that come naturally with the vigorous activities that should be part of our daily living.

The human body is so formed that it must be exercised and exercised correctly in order to remain healthy. Exercise is a much more effective and potent instrument for preserving health when it is more than a haphazard series of movements. With this in mind, Yoga can function as a major factor in the maintenance of your good health, and all the desirable outward appearances of it.

Eugene S. Rawls' and Eve Diskin's book reveals that Yoga is a completely systematized, and yet simple, science of physical conditioning for more healthful living. They further prove the practicality of ancient Yoga for modern people. The practicality of Yoga lies in the fact that its methods work out *every* part of the body, inside and out. There is no age limit for those who can use Yoga successfully. Yoga is easy to learn and simple as well as pleasurable to do.

Exercise is imperative for your good health. Yoga is a splendid and meaningful system to secure and maintain your good health. I highly recommend its regular use.

*D. Richard Sena, M.D.*

# What Yoga Can Do For You

Welcome to the ranks of many thousands who have taken their lives into their own hands.

This book can be your magic key to a new life of glowing health and beauty now *lying dormant within yourself,* waiting to be released—a more wonderful life that can be yours for the taking.

This is the era of the Yoga Revolution. Practically forgotten for centuries, Yoga has emerged to rescue us from the jet-propelled anxieties of our time. Yoga works for everyone. It has become popular with heads of state, stars of films and stage, business men, housewives and students alike.

The rebirth of interest in Yoga has produced a new breed of Woman —Woman as she was meant to be—lovely, relaxed, serene, perennially youthful and, above all, *eternally feminine.* The hazards of modern life have robbed most women of their natural beauty and health birthright, dooming them to fear each approaching year.

No matter what your age, Yoga can be put to work for you. It is never too late to start tapping the rich veins of vitality and beauty lying dormant within every woman.

There is nothing strenuous about Yoga. Every movement is performed slowly, easily, with grace, to prevent the effects of exhaustion which are the enemies of beauty and health. Instead of the aching muscles produced by ordinary "exercise," you experience a delightful *refreshment* of body and spirit which immediately manifests itself in your appearance. Tension is eased without resort to tranquilizers. Skin tone quickly improves. Bodies grown flabby with neglect or disuse take on renewed resilience. All this without fatiguing effort!

There is no "miracle" involved, aside from the one which you will perform yourself with your determination. All of us are born with a potential for a richer life which frequently gets lost in the shuffle as the burdens of fast-paced living descend upon us. What many of us do not recognize is that the chains which prevent us from enjoying good health and knowing true beauty are self-imposed. We have forged them ourselves! Nature never intended life to be a round of migraine, backaches and tranquilizers. We have made ourselves the abject slaves of our own discomfort and lack-lustre appearance. We can, of course, deceive ourselves that we are victims of circumstance. We can waste precious years wallowing in self-pity, or we can take our lives back into our own hands and realize the bounteous reward that Yoga can bring. Without strain you can break the chains that confine the real *you.*

At the very instant you are reading these words, chic and intelligent women your own age—perhaps those you have admired for more years than you like to admit—are refreshing themselves with their Yoga principles. They are recharging their vitalizing batteries of beauty and health so to speak, dissolving the barriers of age distinctions, extending the span of their feminine desirability, bringing forth their true natural beauty which no amount of expensive, cover-up cosmetics nor the most constricting foundation garment can approximate.

A brighter, more meaningful and beautiful life is in your hands with this book. Use its counsel and programs faithfully. You'll be so glad you did!

*Eugene S. Rawls and Eve Diskin*

# ACKNOWLEDGMENTS

We wish to acknowledge the photographic artistry of Robert and Carol Pessak who took all the photographs in this book except the few group photographs.

We also wish to thank the students who posed for the photographs that illustrate Part 5, "Practice Schedules and Special Problems," and we want to express our gratitude to Hildegarde and to Olivia de Havilland for so graciously providing us with photographs of themselves performing the Yoga exercises.

# CONTENTS

# PART ONE

# YOGA –

## for Women

## to Attain

## Lasting Beauty

## and Health

# CHAPTER ONE

# What Is Beauty?

Yoga has a unique viewpoint on the subject of feminine beauty. It maintains

that beauty is an inherent natural attribute of every woman,

that you are in reality beautiful and perfect but that this quality can be concealed, or veiled, by a number of negative conditions that come to reside in you,

that some of these conditions come from the world around you and some come from within,

that the task is not to add beauty to yourself,

that what must be done is to remove the coverings so that your natural perfect beauty will be revealed, and

that the way to remove the negative conditions which veil your true beauty is through the correct practice of Yoga.

In the same way Yoga takes it to be a matter of fact that you are by nature a perfectly healthy person and that, similarly, the job of Yoga is not to make you healthy by *adding* certain qualities to you but is rather to *remove* the conditions that prevent your natural perfect health from manifesting itself and blossoming. It is the contention of Yoga that to the degree that this health is *returned* to you, your inherent beauty automatically shines forth.

Beauty is dependent upon the condition of your health. This includes a healthy state of emotions and mind as well as of the body. Ugly emotions and ugly thoughts cannot be carried in a *truly* beautiful vehicle. Lack of beauty within—anxiety, fear, worry, guilt, envy, hate, vanity— always reveals itself, sooner or later, in the body that carries it. Ultimately, upon attaining the state of real health, physically and mentally, you become your own standard or model of beauty.

Some say that beauty exists only in the eyes of the beholder. (I always ask, what if the beholder has an underdeveloped sense of beauty or none at all?) Other than this point of view, however, we see that a number of supposedly objective standards of beauty exist and we become confused because of the differences in them.

## Standards of Beauty

There are standards of beauty based on what we can call regional taste. What is considered a beautiful woman in France is far different from what is considered a beautiful woman in China or Italy or Senegal or Cuba.

Then there are the standards based on the tastes of different historical eras. Classicists bring forth Greek statues (with accompanying geometrical analyses) to prove that their standard of feminine beauty is the ultimate one. There was the woman of the renaissance. There was the standard of Louis XIV's court. Coming closer to home there was Lillian Russell and her ample hourglass figure which set the style for more than a generation. Then there came the soft, slender, round-shouldered, nearly anemic-looking figure of the pre-World War I era. After that we had the flapper of the twenties, a somewhat athletic type, a hearty Charleston dancing female with her Tom-boyish knees sticking out from under her short, rather comical dress.

Whatever the reason for the ascendency of these concepts of beauty— whether they are imposed upon us by, for example, the clothing and cosmetic industries via Madison Avenue, or whether they are a reflection of unaccountable mass psychological workings within us—we are shackled with our own at the present time.

## The Current Standard of Beauty

Our current public "standard" of feminine beauty has a dual nature. On the one hand there are all the magazines (with corresponding movie stars and entertainment personalities) featuring voluptuous bosomy women with at least 36-24-36 measurements. These are nearly always "men's magazines" and reflect a very large portion of masculine taste.

On the other hand there is the vast ocean of women's magazines and nation-saturating advertisements whose appeal is to women which feature as the criteria of beauty that standard exemplified by the high fashion model. This is (starting from the bottom) a thin-legged, hipless, flat-chested, often skinny-necked female with a pretty though invariably empty face devoid of even the faintest glimmer of character or life. It is a fastidiously made-up shapeless mannequin. This standard—which came about mainly because clothes photograph better on women with this shape—is in the ascendency now and is reaping its devastating effects upon the American public.

Besides the self-evident fact that neither today's high fashion standard nor the Jayne Mansfield type of figure can be considered to be *the* objective standard of feminine beauty, there is a more scientific reason against restricting beauty to the "popular" style of our or any other time. This is the existence of the three basic body types of human beings and all that is implied therein.

## Three Basic Body Types

The three basic body types are the ectomorphic, the mesomorphic and the endomorphic types and are described below:

*The ectomorphic body* is the thin, usually tall, long-legged and somewhat long-waisted type. This includes the average "tall girl."

*The mesomorphic body* corresponds to that which in men would be the muscular athletic type. These are women of medium height, often trim and athletic looking, shapely and full-bodied.

The *endomorphic body* is that which tends to be soft and fat.

We can all point to some extreme example that we know of each type that could well serve as a caricature of that type. We all know the lanky, clumsy beanpole of a woman, or some woman who could pass for an Olympic swimmer. And we all know one or more "fat ladies." What is far more significant, however, is the fact that we can easily find women who represent each of these body types who are beautiful and desirable. Many ectomorphic women are devastating examples of svelte, willowy glamour and beauty. So many mesomorphic women are everything curvaceous and gorgeous. And any number of endomorphic women who, impelled by their own sense of self-respect, have put themselves in proper physical condition are voluptuous and lovely.

## There Is No "Universal Standard" of Beauty

The great lesson in beauty lies here. It is that no one style of beauty can be considered to be *the* universal objective standard. Each woman has to develop her beauty according to her basic body type. Thus women of each type can possess beauty to the most superlative degree and subsequently possess all the joy and natural fulfillment that comes with knowing that their beauty is revealed to its greatest extent.

*Some Specifics on Feminine Beauty*

What then is beauty? Let us answer this question by first listing some of the individual qualities of feminine beauty. These are: good posture, grace of movement, a relaxed carriage, an air of life and vitality, a complexion glowing with natural color, eyes that are bright with life, alertness and interest, a normally firm muscular system, a shape properly proportioned for one's basic bone structure, relaxed features, a calmness of demeanor, and such traits as confidence, friendliness, a sense of humor, lack of vanity and serenity.

These are qualities that can be possessed by every type of woman, from the American farm girl to the New York sophisticate, from the European to the Latin to the Oriental.

Thus another, and by far the most significant question can be asked now. This is: "Are there one or more qualities of beauty that are common denominators running through the examples of beauty from among all the different types of women and which would be considered to be beautiful in all parts of the world and in all different eras?"

The answer is: The characteristics that are common to all types and examples of beauty are the same characteristics that are universally identified with a condition of true health.

If we look at the qualities that are not considered to be beautiful, we will see how (1) these qualities cover up a woman's innate beauty, and, (2) they are symptoms of the lack of a healthful condition.

These non-beautiful characteristics include dull lifeless hair, a tense face, tightness around the lips (the grim-lipped look), lines of tension and fatigue on the face (the drawn look), premature wrinkles around the eyes and the corners of the mouth, a pasty or blemished complexion, double chin, sagging or stringy neck, a sunken chest through poor posture, round-shoulders, the dowager's hump, flabby shapeless upper arms, fat around the waist, a pot belly, excess weight and flab around the hips, shapeless oversized buttocks, shapeless overweight thighs, a graceless walk, lack of general bodily poise, a look of anxiety and tension, a stiff inflexible bearing, nervous jerky movements, talking too fast through nervousness, the gaunt semi-emaciated look of a woman who has subjected herself to excessive dieting (on the assumption that because fat is ugly, thinness in itself is beautiful), and an obvious absence of the self-confidence that a serene mind brings.

*Awaking All Your Dormant Beauty*

Now we can see the basic principle behind this book; that is, *beauty is dormant within you*. It is covered by one or a number of negative conditions. (All non-beautiful characteristics are cured by removal, not by adding a quality of beauty in their place as if that quality did not already exist in you.) Achieving a state of true health is the only way to remove such negative factors and reveal your real beauty which has lain covered up.

The science of Hatha Yoga removes these negative conditions from your body. It also prevents them from returning or from arriving in the first place. Nothing can do more to prevent your falling out of shape than a fifteen or twenty minute session of Yoga each day.

The state of health that Yoga brings automatically reveals your natural beauty. This means a relaxed face with its subsequent soft lips and pleasant look, a superlative complexion, smooth and glowing, a graceful firm neck, a well developed chest through lovely posture, a shapely back, a slim waist, an abdomen correctly flat for your body type, firm shapely hips, firm and correctly proportioned buttocks, taut sleek thighs, an easy grace, poise, an air of relaxation, calmness and self-confidence, and many other wonderful, normal characteristics which you were meant to have by nature.

Thus we see the perfectly geared relationship of Yoga to health and health to beauty. Proper physical, emotional and mental condition reveals a depth of beauty that can easily override the lack of one or another specific attribute of beauty. The woman whose nose is a bit long, whose chin recedes slightly, or who may be too tall or by the nature of her body type and bone structure have too ample a hip spread can, without the slightest difficulty, be beautiful, alluring and attractive by putting herself in her best physical condition and by possessing the traits of emotional and mental health that come with the practice of Yoga.

## How Yoga Brings Grace to Beauty

Webster says that beauty is "an assemblage of graces or properties which command the approbation of the senses; those qualities which are most pleasing to the eye." Yoga would amend his definition slightly by adding that beauty appeals to more than the eye and strikes a chord within man that goes deeper than the senses alone. Many a man has seen "an assemblage of graces that commanded the approbation of his senses" only to approach a little closer or let a little time pass and realize with disappointment that what he saw was a superficial, unreal beauty; a mask.

When a woman is in the healthful condition that reveals her inherent loveliness, she is far more likely to possess the emotional stability and mental peace which complete her beauty. These higher traits are brought about by Yoga along with a condition of supreme physical health and fitness.

# CHAPTER TWO

# Beauty Through Health

The health problems of modern women are mainly responsible for their beauty problems. Tension, overweight, nerves, fatigue and all the rest, whatever their ultimate causes, result in the disintegration of a woman's appearance and the covering up of her natural inherent beauty. *Fatigue* gives a woman a drawn, washed-out look. *Tension* produces lines of strain. *Overweight* results in a distortion of various major areas of the body (hips, buttocks, thighs, abdomen, waist) and the rendering of what nature intended to be a normal and lovely creature into something grotesque. And so it goes, all the way down the line.

The modern woman needs a practical, efficient means of coping with these health problems, a method that will both overcome the existing problems and prevent them from reappearing. Most of the methods known today do nothing but force some pounds off usually in an exhausting, boring and time-consuming manner. No system of exercise can compare to the science of Hatha Yoga for banishing tension (no matter how deep rooted), nervousness, excess poundage, chronic fatigue and all the rest. Hatha Yoga is the most efficient, time-saving and effortless method known to put you in the absolute peak of fitness and health so that you can enjoy the blessings of life and health and the superlative appearance that comes with such a state.

## How Yoga Banishes Tension

Tension is a condition that has reached proportions of being a chronic national malady. One characteristic of tension is a tightening and constricting of the body. The most familiar locations are the small muscles of the neck and the great trapezius muscle that stretches from the neck to the shoulders. Many other areas are victims of tension to an equal or less obvious degree. This tightening results in pain and discomfort. In the long run it distorts the posture and contributes to the premature and unnatural stiffening of the entire body.

The stiffness and inflexibility of the body which comes from tension is in itself the cause of dangerous physical conditions. Even the stiffness which is obvious in the physical organisms of elderly people is in the eyes of Yoga an absolutely unnatural and unnecessary condition. This inflexibility of the body is so much more unnatural and dangerous to the health when it appears, as it now nearly universally does, in the bodies of younger people. The average person of thirty today is nearly as stiff and inelastic physically as the person of sixty.

The cause of tension is twofold. All those causes of tension with which we are most familiar and which come from the world around us are secondary causes. These include personal relations with people, problems on the job, worries about the future, social pressure, keeping up with the Joneses (and everything involved in that absurd compulsion), the harsh nerve-shattering noise of modern city life with its automobiles and roaring airplanes, the pace that kills, the devastating lack of beauty of so much of our surroundings, and that ever-present bugbear of modern life, the world situation with its storehouse of fuel to keep our every anxiety aflame, ranging from the atom bomb to wars in various parts of our planet.

As real as these matters are that give rise to tension, to the Yogi they are nonetheless classified as secondary causes. The primary cause of tension exists always and only within the individual human being. For when a person has become aware of the primary cause of tension within himself and has dealt with it correctly and overcome it, all the secondary causes, from your mother-in-law to the bills piling up on the kitchen table to the threat of atomic war, are no longer able to produce the slightest nuance of fear, anxiety or worry. It is then that Yoga deals with and overcomes the primary cause of tension. A detailed description of the actual "cause within" is treated in the section on *Beauty and Health Through Peace of Mind*.

The Yoga method of overcoming tension and all the problems that come with it is by employing its time-honored and proven physical and mental techniques. The mind, however insubstantial an organism it is to us, is dealt with directly by means of the mental exercises of Raja Yoga. First, however, the student must become accustomed to the method of using Yoga and at the same time must remove the tension from his physical body by means of Hatha Yoga. The body is so much more available to our direct control than the mind that it is logical to first gain the immediate, positive results of the physical exercises.

The Yogic method of overcoming stiffness consists of the ingenious, scientific stretching postures. These postures stretch every portion of the body from toe to neck and face, and restore the original flexibility and limberness which you had in your earliest youth.

This new-found physical flexibility and relaxation results in an immediate and exquisitely delightful relief from tension. It results in the freeing of an enormous quantity of natural energy, the life-force, which was hitherto trapped in those various tense areas.

## How Slim Should You Really Be?

What is both desirable and necessary is to be at the trimmest weight for your body type. In the case of an ectomorph, this can be quite thin. Katharine Hepburn, in her prime, could become as thin as she wanted and look more charming for every pound less. Women of the other body types, though, should retain the curves natural to their basic form. If these women reduce past a certain weight, they will invariably come to possess the familiar "forced" slender look which is a detriment to beauty.

In any case, your beauty will be brought out to perfection according to your natural capabilities if you reach *your* natural weight and *your* best physical condition by means of Yoga. If you develop your health and bring out your beauty this way, you will never look like an old woman who is desperately (and pathetically) *trying* to look young. You will never look like a shapely woman who has neurotically starved herself into the form she had "once" at the age of fifteen.

My first advice to women who have chosen a degree of slimness to which they aspire is to be sure that the motive behind your desire is not one of emotional insecurity. How little faith one must have in oneself to be unable to face the fact that you are thirty-five. And the irony of it is that when a woman is in her best physical condition, the years as such cannot have a detrimental effect upon the degree of her loveliness, beauty and charm. There is a vast difference between the normal healthy female self-respect which makes a woman want to be feminine and attractive at any age, and the pride of a woman who wishes only to keep deceiving herself into thinking that she can always look twenty.

My second piece of advice is for you to remember that slimness is necessary only to the extent that it corresponds to your basic bodily structure.

This concept then leaves out all unnatural or quick weight-reducing methods. The slimness you will attain through Yoga will be pleasant to come by, of a very long lasting nature, and will make your weight and shape correspond to your natural body type.

## *The Use of Sun and Air*

So many women who complain of beauty problems spend their leisure time in activities that are not conducive to bringing about beauty or health. *Your leisure is the time to do something that will augment your health, beauty, long life and peace of mind.*

We have lost so very much of man's normal closeness to nature and the results are devastating. Tens upon tens of millions of people are truly "closed in" against the natural world around them. To contrast this with a people who have retained a closeness to nature, in Japan nearly all houses have sliding walls that open into gardens or natural vistas or at least the open air. The outside is considered as much a part of the home as that segment of nature which can be temporarily surrounded by walls. How many people even sit in their backyards, much less eat in them when the weather permits. A cookout is a big occasion, a self-conscious affair, virtually a celebration when in reality it could and should be a normal customary habit for more than six months out of the year.

The harm lies in the fact that nature possesses healing and regenerative powers. Actually nothing else does. When you are ill, it is the natural forces in your body that make the body cure itself. Nothing is truer than the old saying that the doctor only helps nature cure you. Exposure and acclimatization to the world of nature has extraordinary powers to build and rebuild health and to soothe and heal us both physically and mentally.

What is essential is to immerse yourself as much as possible in the healing rejuvenating world of nature. This means walk instead of ride at every possible occasion. If you do not live directly in the heart of a metropolis such as Manhattan, get a bicycle and use it. Make it part of your life. Ride it on every short or fairly short errand you have to do. If the bank is too far to walk to, use a bicycle. Use it for shopping as much as you can. Your health, now and in the future, is what is involved. Live vigorously.

You cannot get too much fresh air. It rejuvenates you, replenishes your vitality and energy, heals you and makes you hardy. It gives you the feeling of being fully alive.

The sun is also a primary source of health and beauty. Practice a bit of moderation in regard to the sun, however. The deep mahogany tan or the leathery hide is not necessarily the best thing to have in many cases. Nothing, however, makes you feel so wonderfully full of life as a suntan, and nothing is so lovely as beautifully tanned skin.

It does not have to be the summer vacation suntan. Exposure to the brisk outdoors of autumn or the beautiful stimulation of winter in the woods or along the shore gives the face a rosy, delightful and absolutely lovely glow of health and natural color.

Use the sun and air not as pleasant "occasions" but to such an extent that they are a very important part of your life. You should become so habituated to sun and fresh air that you miss them and crave them—like a famished person craves food—if you do not have them for a few hours.

## *Beauty Through Yoga, Peace and Right Attitude*

As we have stated, nothing shows so obviously on a person's exterior than the sum total of his or her habitual emotional pattern. Remember, however, your good emotions will always outshine your negative feelings.

This cannot be faked. The ability of a woman to "think herself beautiful" in a mechanical fashion is extremely limited. By mechanical I refer to such a method as repeating to oneself over and over, "Every day in every way I get better and better." The simple fact of the matter is that while the repeating of that phrase might perk you up somewhat in the beginning, you can repeat it from now until doomsday and you will *not* get better and better in every way.

Nothing shines so on the outside than inner peace of mind, heart and spirit. This is revealed by gentleness, kindness, compassion, even-temperedness, good-naturedness, calm, repose, serenity, good humor, poise, grace, a clear lovely expression in the eyes, a smooth complexion and a considerable list of similar attributes. Therefore it is necessary not only to attain a modicum of peace but, even from the beginning, to have a right attitude toward beauty, health, people and life.

The right attitude toward health includes the following notions: health is an uppermost necessity and *must* be possessed; health is to be had by means of a correct method; in order to have health, the individual cannot sit back and wait for it to automatically develop but must take the matter in hand and do something active to bring it about; and, the individual needs to realize that you only receive to the degree in which you are willing to give in terms of interest, determination and action.

The right attitude to beauty must include the ideas that: true beauty exists within you; it is your unique birthright; the beauty you manifest must be genuine and not a facsimile forced or applied from the outside; real beauty is unself-conscious; and, the beauty you reveal has to be the result of a healthy, strong, confident way of life.

If you have a right attitude, not only toward the attainment of beauty but toward life and people, your natural beauty will reveal itself directly in proportion to how few so-called imperfections yet veil it. Hatha Yoga then automatically removes those beauty-concealing and health hazardous imperfections (overweight, stiffness, etc.). The state of peace, developed so efficiently by the mental exercises of Raja Yoga, makes the physical transfiguration complete.

Yoga is an active, self-performed step toward health and real inner peace. The by-products of health and peace come automatically, including beauty of appearance, happiness, calmness of spirit, strength of character and all the numerous other attributes discussed in detail in forthcoming chapters.

# CHAPTER THREE

# What Is HATHA YOGA?

The word Yoga is the name of the science of physical and mental deveolpment that originated in the land of India many centuries ago. It is an exact science whose purpose is to bring the body into a state of unexcelled physical health and well-being and to bring to the mind peace and serenity in the midst of the problems and pressures of everyday living.

## Hatha and Raja Yoga

The science of Yoga is divided into two main parts. These are Hatha Yoga and Raja Yoga. Hatha Yoga is in itself a complete science. It deals with the physical body and is the form of Yoga with which people are most familiar. The science of Hatha Yoga consists of three basic kinds of exercises. These are (1) cleansing techniques, (2) postures, and, (3) breathing exercises.

## Cleansing Techniques

The cleansing techniques are designed to remove harmful impurities from various internal parts of the body. One of the cleansing techniques that is taught in this book cleans and purifies the lungs of many impurities that have come to lodge in them through the breathing of toxic fumes and from the smoking of cigarettes. All cleansing techniques have wonderful side effects in addition to their purifying ability. This technique, *The Cleans-*

*ing Breath,* is a tremendous strengthener of the lung tissue itself. There is another cleansing technique taught in this book called *The Abdominal Contraction* which is of such profound importance to the health of the human body that I have devoted an entire chapter to it. This ingenious body movement promotes and guarantees normal regularity. It has had amazing results in breaking nearly lifelong laxative addiction. It is, in fact, the only natural method known to man for the regaining of normal natural regularity. The *Abdominal Contraction* also massages, stimulates and improves the circulation in numerous vital internal organs upon which true health and long life depend. Another of its side effects is to firm and reduce excess weight in the abdomen.

## Postures

The second kind of exercise that comes under the science of Hatha Yoga are the postures. The postures (asanas, in Sanskrit) are just what the name implies. They are positions into which you place and hold your body. These positions enable your body to bring about certain remarkable healthful changes, improvements which both eliminate and prevent negative conditions.

The postures are the physical exercises with which people are generally more familiar and which have come to be identified with Yoga. There are three varieties of Yoga postures. They are (1) *stretching postures,* (2) *inversion postures,* and, (3) *sitting postures.*

The *stretching postures* consist of a limited number of nearly effortless scientific stretches of the body. The muscles, ligaments and tendons are the first parts to receive the benefits of stretching. These tissues have, in nearly all people, grown tight through nervous tension and other unnatural causes. Wherever such tightness exists in the body, your energy and vitality is being drained and lost. Stretching these muscles, ligaments and tendons to their normal natural resiliency results in a state of profound relaxation and a freedom from accumulated tension.

While making these tissues flexible has healthful and relaxing effects upon your body, you are also taking a step toward normalizing the condition of your spinal column. The greatest emphasis in Hatha Yoga is on restoring, by exact scientific stretching, the natural condition of the spine which is one of great flexibility and elasticity.

In Hatha Yoga the spinal column is carefully, methodically and scientifically stretched in its four basic directions: forward, backward, in a spiral or twisting direction, and sideway. The complete limberness that the spine was meant by nature to have is attained through this method. Many people are amazed by the flexibility and limberness attained by means of Hatha Yoga. What people should be amazed at, however, is the rigidity and stiffness that nearly everyone's body has come to possess due to our debilitating modern way of life, in contrast to the natural healthy state of man.

As lovely and enjoyable as this limberness is, the results of it are what are important to you. The first result is that you feel and look years younger. It brings about deep relaxation, increased vitality and a strong healthy nervous system. Numerous other results are described and explained in detail in the exercise portion of this book. The stretching postures of Hatha Yoga also adjust the spinal column vertebra by vertebra and are equivalent to the Yoga student receiving a mild and gentle chiropractic spinal adjustment every day.

In the *inversion postures,* the body is turned upside-down and held that way for a short while. The two most important and well-known of these inversion postures are taught in this book. They are *The Shoulder Stand* and *The Head Stand.* The healthful effects are tremendous. They help reduce weight, improve the complexion, rest various internal organs, stimulate vital glands, and refresh the brain (with a subsequent increase of mental alertness and clarity). The way the inversion postures accomplish all their marvelous results is by improving the circulation of blood throughout the entire body. This is not the superficial stimulation of circulation that is provided by ordinary exercise in which the heart is temporarily caused to pump strenuously, but an improvement of circulation that is of a profound and long lasting nature. At the same time it is brought about in an effortless, motionless manner, making it perfectly suitable for people of all ages and for persons who are simply not interested any more in putting themselves through the grueling and discouraging rigors of strenuous exercise.

The *sitting postures* consist of a few simple, ancient sitting positions which calm the metabolism, tranquilize the nerves and help replenish your vitality. The sitting postures also work well in combination with the breathing exercises of Yoga.

## Breathing Exercises

Breathing exercises are the third basic category of Hatha (physical) Yoga techniques and certainly deserve their legendary fame. While part of the science of Hatha Yoga, the Yoga breathing exercises are in themselves a separate science which in India is called "Pranayama." Prana means "life-force" or that power which animates all living things. Yama means "control." And so the science of Yogic breathing was originally called "control of the life-force." The implications here are most profound and should be of interest to anyone who wishes to live a long, full and healthy life.

The Yoga breathing exercises are simple, natural, wholesome and immensely healthful. The three basic exercises of the Yogic science of breathing are taught in this book. Some of the results of their practice are: relaxation and calming of the nervous system, improved sleep, the overcoming of insomnia, development and strengthening of the lungs, purifying the blood itself (through increased oxygen intake), development of the chest cavity and diaphragm, increased energy and vitality, the overcoming of fatigue, a lovely complexion, and the glow of generally improved health.

## Raja Yoga

Raja Yoga is that branch of Yoga which deals directly with the mind. Like Hatha Yoga, it is a complete science in itself. Raja Yoga is the world renowned science of mind control and consists of a small number of mental exercises that are designed to calm and quiet the agitated mind. These exercises are simple, natural and delightful to practice and have far-reaching results in terms of emotional and mental health. A full explanation of the Yogic science of mind control and two of the mental exercises are given in the section on *Beauty and Health Through Peace of Mind*.

The "mind control" we speak of is that which renders the mind the efficient servant of man rather than the frequently irresponsible and in many instances tyrannical master it has come to be. The ultimate result of the practice of Raja (mental) Yoga is the banishing from our lives of such unnecessary burdens as anxiety, worry, fear, guilt, insecurity and anger, and bringing to the individual true and lasting serenity of mind.

# CHAPTER FOUR

# How to Evaluate
# Your Beauty Problem

Joseph Conrad said: "No man ever understands quite his own artful dodges to escape from the grim shadow of self-knowledge." Absolute or complete self-knowledge from the Yogic point of view is, however, not a grim shadow but is rather *the* ultimate illuminating and glorious experience of which a human being is capable. In the beginning , however, in the first stages of the path to self-knowledge, those first insights or honest appraising looks at oneself can be grim, depressing or even shocking in some cases. The path of self-development requires a high level of honesty and courage.

Your first objective tool in this task is your mirror. According to the degree of your honesty and courage, your mirror can be your best friend or a hateful enemy. The mirror never really lies. Only your own "artful dodges" can deceive you when you stand before it and begin your questioning. Only you can ask the questions. And only you can answer them. (Very few people are fortunate enough to have had another person present them with the questions and answers and fewer are able to withstand having others see their imperfections without resistance and resentment.)

Go into your room. Lock the door. You are with yourself . . . alone. This deliberate solitude, this conscious action of self-examination, is something woefully lacking in our modern lives, so under the spell are we of the hypnotic effect of activity. No matter what our particular use of this time of introspection, it is something we need desperately in our lives if we are to talk of mental health or dare to dream of peace of mind.

Remove every stitch of clothing and then . . . go stand in front of your mirror. Hardly a woman alive has not looked into a mirror and counted imperfections, minor ones when young, more frightening ones when the year of thirty has passed. But now for the first time, be professional about this look. No more careless, haphazard, self-deceiving perusals: now look and inquire in an exhaustive dedicated way. Do not allow any emotions whatever to arise during this period. This is to be a cold calculating appraisal. Look at yourself with the eyes of a beauty connoisseur and with the eyes of all the people who see you in life, both men and women.

## Your Check List of Obvious Questions

Here are some of the more obvious questions you should ask.

1. What do I want out of life that relates to or depends upon my physical appearance?
2. Is my present physical appearance a help or a hindrance to the attaining of my desires?
3. How deeply is my beauty buried beneath negative conditions?
4. Do I have one outstanding appearance problem? If so, what is it?
5. Where is my first major problem area?
   (a) Above the shoulders?
   (b) Between my shoulders and hips?
   (c) From my hips down?
6. What *general* improvement do I need first?
7. What beauty problem of mine is easiest to overcome?
8. What problem area on me is most easily improved?
9. What specific improvements do I need?
   (a) Is my face (excessively wrinkled for my age) (tense and strained) (blotched) (pasty) (sagging) (pudgy) (tired)?
   (b) Is my neck (sagging) (stringy) (lacking in muscle tone) (double-chinned) (wrinkled)?
   (c) Is my back (matronly) (held poorly posturewise)?
   (d) Is my chest (underdeveloped) (sunken through poor posture or other reasons)?
   (e) Are my arms (flabby) (skinny) (fat) (weak)?
   (f) Is my waist (fat) (shapeless)?
   (g) Is my abdomen (flabby) (fat) (protruding due to bad posture)?
   (h) Are my hips (overweight) (skinny) (flabby)?
   (i) Are my buttocks (sagging) (overweight)?
   (j) Are my thighs (flabby) (wrinkled) (fat)?

(k) Are my feet (misshapen) (ugly)?

10. What *sensible* model should I choose to be the standard that I will strive to attain through Yoga?

11. Do I look alive and vital or apathetic and depressed?

12. Have I a nervous appearance?

13. What nervous habits do I have that mar my beauty? (Nail biting, fidgeting, twiddling my fingers, compulsive foot-tapping, incessant chattering, eye blinking, talking too loud, fast movements.)

14. Have I a soothing or an irritating effect on people?

15. Are my movements generally graceful?

16. Have I sufficient poise?

17. Is my appearance truly feminine or do I have a "hard look" to me?

18. Do I appear self-confident or of low personal self-sufficiency?

19. Is my demeanor friendly or defensive?

20. Do I hold myself proudly (but without vanity) like a beautiful woman should?

21. Is my posture correct and contributing to my best appearance?

22. How much weight should I lose in order to satisfy *myself?* (Estimate this sensibly. Choose a realistic attainable goal. Forget the charts on the public scales or in the magazines. If the chart says you should lose twenty pounds, ask yourself what you would look like if you lost ten and whether you are capable of taking and keeping off that much.)

23. What are my best points regarding physical beauty?

24. Have I been living a mole-like life, unexposed to the beauty-giving elements of sun and fresh air?

Answer these questions honestly and to the best of your ability. Then, based on your answers, begin practicing the wonderfully rejuvenating exercises taught in this book, adhering as close as you can to the instructions and to the practice schedule (in the section *Practice Schedules*) that applies closest to your main beauty problems.

CHAPTER FIVE

# What the Yoga Exercises Can Do for You

With each exercise taught in this book, a complete analysis is given of what that particular exercise does for your body. The results of these exercises have been proven by (1) millions of people just like yourself who have practiced them for over fifty centuries, (2) hundreds of thousands of people in our own time, from every walk of life and in every civilized country on earth, who practice them, and (3) modern medical investigation.

## Beauty Benefits of Daily Yoga Practice

Here are a number of the general effects that a moderate daily practice of Yoga will have upon you.

*Relief from Tension.* Tension is locked in the tight stiffened areas of your body. The Yoga exercises stretch these areas loose while restoring your youthful limberness. At the same time they release the tension from such areas as the neck, the back, the spine, etc.

*Normalized Weight.* There is no better way to reduce than by means of the Yoga techniques because weight lost through Yoga tends to stay off.

*A Trim and Firm Figure.* While the inversion exercises in combination with the stretching exercises removes excess weight, the stretches give you vibrant muscle tone and make your body trim, firm and sleek.

19

*Rejuvenation of Sagging Face and Neck Muscles.* There are specific Yoga exercises that deal directly with the face and neck. By means of these particular techniques the muscles of the neck and face that have begun to sag through lack of use and improper circulation are reconditioned and "perked up" into splendid and more youthful condition.

*Improvement of Your Complexion.* Here again the wonderful way in which Yoga brings increased circulation to what are usually nourishment-starved areas of the body results in a glowing complexion full of color. The relaxation and relief from chronic tension also contributes much to a delightfully improved complexion.

*Your Lungs Become Cleansed and Strengthened.* This is a result *that money cannot buy.* There is no price on healthy lungs in this age of smog, fallout, cigarette smoke, insecticides and toxic machine fumes. The Yoga breathing exercises taught in this book purify and strengthen the lung tissue.

*Circulation Improved.* This is a major function of Yoga. Circulation is gently improved by means of the stretching exercises and is driven home with the inversion techniques, The Head Stand and The Shoulder Stand. This is not a superficial effect but a deep and complete improvement of bodily circulation that includes all the internal organs.

*The Brain Is Refreshed.* We tend to take the brain for granted as an internal organ. We rarely if ever think of it in terms of "physical" fatigue or wear and tear. Yet the fact is that because of the heart's difficulty in circulating blood throughout every portion of the body above the neck, the brain is in a majority of instances starved for the nourishment and vitality that it is the job of proper blood circulation to bring. The Yoga exercises scientifically increase the circulation in the brain itself. This refreshes that organ and results in a greater awareness and alertness. There is nothing more wonderful for the entire nervous system.

*Overcome Chronic Fatigue.* The effect of Yoga upon the brain also results in the overcoming of that chronic fatigue which settles upon a person and which is to a very great extent due to lack of sufficient circulation in this vital area. The tension-removing, energizing and revitalizing effect of the stretching exercises gives a new endurance that also does away with the life-draining fatigue that plagues so many modern people.

*Calm Nerves.* Nothing can so calm the nerves as Yoga. First the body is relieved of accumulated tension by means of the stretching postures. These same postures strengthen and calm the nerves while the breathing exercises complete the task. One of the overall effects of practicing Yoga daily, and according to a correct schedule, is the acquisition of calmness, repose and serenity.

*Increased Emotional Control.* This is not the emotional control that comes from the false path of "bottling up" the emotions or repressing them through a forceful or artificial discipline which is not conducive to emotional and mental health. I refer to the calm and equanimity that comes. from a healthy nervous system and a healthy state of mind. The Alternate Nostril Breathing Exercise alone has the ability to calm upset emotions at any time.

*The Ability to Be Relaxed in Any Circumstance.* The Yogi is not blown here and there emotionally like a leaf before the wind of aggravating circumstances. Events of life can rage around you like a storm but you will remain a calm untroubled point within it through Yoga. This is not apathy but is rather a state of higher awareness and control over conditions that are much too far beneath you to warrant your becoming upset. The relaxation is really a newfound mastery of life.

*Improved Sleep.* This is axiomatic. There are specific exercises designed to overcome any sleep problem and to make your night's rest the healing beautifying experience it should be.

*Abundant Energy and Vitality.* The student of Yoga will observe an immediate increase in physical endurance. This is the result of the marvelous vitality that comes with the practice of Yoga. It is not a "new" vitality, however; it is simply the making available to you that which has always been yours by nature but which was being drained away from you by all the tension that accumulated in your body. Your new energy is something which you will experience very strongly. It is a "life" and vitality which is also felt by other people and the "verve" spoken of in all writings on beauty.

*Youthful Limberness.* Naturally, the first thing that happens to you in Yoga is that you become limber, flexible and elastic. The restoration of this quality of youth is indeed like a physical rebirth. It is a nearly ineffable release from the bondage of the tightening and stiffening that characterizes the arrival of premature age. People sense something "new and different" about you.

*Vital Glands and Organs Are Stimulated.* The immensity of this area can barely be introduced here. Health is in reality an internal matter. All external characteristics of health (such as beauty, for example) are but the outward signs of an inner state of being. The Yoga exercises improve the condition of your most vital internal glands and organs. These are what keep you going. If they function as nature meant them to, then you stride through a life in which your body is indeed the temple of the spirit and reveals itself as such. The Yoga exercises actually reach into your body and bring about specific improvements in specific internal parts such as the heart, the brain, the lungs, the colon, the thyroid gland, the kidneys and others.

*Resistance to Common Disorders.* You will find, when you practice Yoga for a while, that you are no longer susceptible to colds, headaches and other such common complaints as you were before.

*A Radiant Appearance.* All the foregoing effects contribute to bringing out your beauty to a degree commensurate with how correctly, regularly and sincerely you practice. The calm serenity, the air of relaxation, the grace, the poise and the vitality (among other traits) that you come to have through the practice of Yoga result in the radiance of a person whose potential beauty manifests itself in every movement.

# CHAPTER SIX

# Is Age a Bar to
# Yoga Practice?

The answer is unequivocally "NO." No one is too old to practice Yoga. I myself have had much experience teaching Yoga to senior citizens both in my public classes and in homes for elderly people. I have had one class in which the *average* age was seventy-three. One of the most wonderful and revealing things about Yoga is the incredible range of humanity who can practice it and receive its results.

## Why School Children and Students Need Yoga

School children can practice Yoga and would do well to do so. It builds the health of young people and takes the edge off the restless emotions of youth, being calming and maturing. High school and college students should by all means practice Yoga. Besides the physical benefits, nothing can enable the young man or young woman to study so well. It clears the mind, increases endurance, calms the restless nervous system and develops the powers of concentration.

## How Yoga Helps in Sports

Athletes of the hardiest types reap great benefits from Yoga. I had a professional prize-fighter in my class who later told me that his practice of Yoga increased his ability in the ring. It gave him greater control over

his nerves and his breath. The average person from thirty to fifty constitutes a major portion of Yoga students. These people need a form of
physical culture that is simple, interesting, non-strenuous and which does
not take much time to practice. When we come to people who are at the
end of middle age and beyond, most of us somehow or other presume that
they will have no interest in or need for physical exercise except perhaps
shuffleboard or golf in the case of a long-time golf enthusiast.

## Urgent Need for Older People to Practice Yoga Exercises

The fact is that the older a person is the more urgently he or she
needs correct exercise. So many of my students of mature years inform
me that they began Yoga because their doctor *ordered* them to exercise
"or else." The person who "sits down" when she reaches a certain age and
thinks she doesn't need to be physically active in the sense of genuine
exercise is to a very great extent committing slow suicide. This is because
it is the nature of the human body to fall slowly apart from non-use. It is
a law of nature that the parts of the human body must be used, and used
correctly, or they will deteriorate.

While it is easy to understand the necessity for people to exercise
at every age level, what must be determined is what kind of exercise is
available and proper for an average person over forty. It must be a system
of exercise that works out all the parts of the body. It must be a system
the difficulty of which can be varied to correspond with the individual's
limitations. It must be a system involving gentle exercises. Yoga possesses
all these attributes.

An athletic person can go at Yoga in such a manner as to suit her
robust nature and constitution. The most fragile older citizen can practice a full Yoga exercise schedule in such a manner as to suit perfectly
her mild requirements. Yoga can be tuned down, so to speak, to suit
any physical makeup.

Yet, as gently as older persons might practice Yoga, they receive
enormous benefits from it. They do become more limber—amazingly so. I
have had an *eighty*-year-old gentleman in my class who, in the course of
one year, became more flexible than the average forty-year-old. They reap
all the benefits to the nerves, to the heart, to the circulation, and on top
of the obvious physical benefits, to the morale and the spirit. Nothing can
keep one so full of life, spirit and a feeling of well-being as Yoga.

The capabilities of the body and mind are not in nature limited by
age. Only wrong living habits or neglect deteriorate the body and mind
to the tragic and pathetic extent which we see around us every day. For
example, in the mental realm we can point to Bertrand Russell, Albert
Schweitzer, Einstein, Eleanor Roosevelt and a host of other world notables

who in very old age made mockeries of the average younger person in terms of physical and mental energy, leadership, creativity, brilliance, and contribution to the betterment of mankind.

In the physical realm we can point to people of mature years whose physical attributes were nothing short of phenomenal. We all know of the eternal beauty, vivacity and talent of such women as Marlene Dietrich and Gloria Swanson (who practices Yoga regularly as part of her way of life). There was Bernard MacFadden, the world famous health authority, who, in his seventies, would parachute out of airplanes. Mr. Mikume of Japan is the world Judo master at the age of seventy-five. And in Japan also, Mr. Moribei Uyishiba, at ninety-five hurls *four and five* black belt Judo champions around at once as if they were children. These men can work out with young and competitive Judo champions for hours and not even lose their breath. You have doubtless seen instances of this seemingly eternal vigor and youth in persons of mature years.

In Yoga, a person's real age has very little to do with how many years they have lived. I know people who are young at sixty and seventy, and I know people who are old at thirty. I have known college students who were old in demeanor, attitude and outlook, and who, if they were seen in silhouettes, would more often than not be considered to be physically old as well. Their bodies were flabby. They had a paunch. Their muscles were soft and without tone. Their shoulders were round, their posture sagging and they walked without life and vitality. Surely this is age.

What then gives some people the quality of youth and the ability to retain it despite the years? And what is it that, conversely, deprives many a young person of this quality and gives him the aspect of age and decrepitude? There is no doubt that some people are simply gifted by nature with a constitution and a metabolism that enables them to remain vigorous and youthful of appearance on into their later years. These instances, however, are unusual exceptions. The general rule is that proper *use* of the body results in the retention of the characteristics of youth. The essence of *proper use* of the body has been systematized in the science of Hatha Yoga.

## Yoga Always Works

One of the aspects of Yoga that makes it so welcome and successful in the West is the logic of it. A certain bodily movement is performed and a certain effect must consistently take place. Yet with all its incontrovertible logic and its proven ability to overcome tremendous obstructions and to produce health, many people looked puzzled when confronted with the statement that it *always* works.

This is because the modern western mind has a negative reaction to the notion of perfection. Perfection is supposed to be some kind of impossibility. Everything can be improved.

The fact remains that Yoga has been used and tested by millions of people for over fifty centuries and not only has it always lived up to its claims but in all that time no improvement has been able to be made on it. Nothing has had to be taken away and nothing has had to be added. The reason is simple—it is a perfected system. Except for instances of major illness or physical disability, Yoga *always* works.

If you place your body in a Yoga posture and move correctly as instructed, your body *must stretch*. If you manipulate your body as instructed, certain specific effects *must and always will* take place. There is no "hit or miss" in Yoga.

The power of Yoga is enormous. You may be so stiff that in bending forward your hands can't even reach your knees, but if you practice the Yoga exercises correctly, according to the instructions in this book, you will find that, inevitably as day must follow night, your stiffened body (back, spine, legs, tendons, ligaments, muscles) will "give" and you will experience the thrill of seeing your flexibility increase a little more each day. In a very short time you will be as limber and elastic of body as you were half a lifetime ago.

I have used the regaining of flexibility as one example of how no human organism can withstand the methodical scientific stretching techniques of Yoga. All other healthful results come about just as inevitably. Besides the mechanical perfection of the science of Yoga, the subconscious intelligence residing in both body and mind wishes very much for these beneficial results to take place and contributes its power to help bring them about.

# CHAPTER SEVEN

# How to Practice Yoga

The first step is to set the correct scene as much as you are able. Try to practice in a place that is conducive toward your performing the exercises in a leisurely way. It is best to be alone in a room so that you can concentrate fully upon what you are doing. The room should be quiet. The freer your practice time is from such distractions as children running around, the better will be your results. Make sure that the room is well ventilated. The more fresh air available to you during your practice period the more benefit you will obtain.

Dress in a comfortable manner so that you can stretch and move about freely. Shorts, a bathing suit, leotards, or a loose light garment like a "muu-muu" are all quite suitable.

Make sure that the surface is not too soft. You don't want to practice on anything like a bed or mattress or excessively thick foam rubber mat. On surfaces such as these your body will tend to sink in and you will be unable to assume the positions correctly. This will deprive you of much of their benefit. Nor of course should you practice on, for example, a hard terrazzo floor where the discomfort might discourage you or shorten your workout. A normal thick carpet is good or a couple of blankets doubled over with perhaps a smooth straw mat on top.

## Be Relaxed Always with Yoga

It is important, as much as you are able, to approach your practice period with a serene state of mind. Leave all hurry behind. Remember the importance of this brief period of time that you are taking out of the day. The purpose of this time is of great significance to your life. Resolve to use it in a relaxed unhurried manner.

Do everything you can to practice at approximately the same time every day. Don't be a martinet: that is, forcing yourself to be on the spot at exactly the stroke of five each afternoon. You should, however, definitely pick the time of day that is best for you, such as late morning, late afternoon, or early evening, and then tend to practice at that time regularly. You will find that regularity of practice brings the best results.

The length of your workout will depend partially on how long you have been practicing Yoga. At first you will be holding a posture for a very short time, usually ten seconds. As time passes, and you add the few required seconds each week and your interest and enthusiasm builds as it invariably does, you may find that you are capable of enjoying a longer workout. At that stage the length of your daily workout will depend on the time limitations of your daily schedule. In general, however, you should be able to get maximum results from as little as twenty minutes of practice each day. The most important thing is to stick to a regular, methodical pattern and to follow the carefully planned practice schedules in the book.

The first key to success in the practice of Yoga is *Slow-Motion*. Only through slow-motion are all the wonderful benefits attained. It is the slowness of movement that produces depth, strength and long-lasting results. You must move slowly, as if in a dream. For example, in bending forward at the waist from a standing position, you should take a minimum of ten full seconds from the time that you begin your forward movement to the time you are down as far as you can go. You will enjoy the slow-motion aspect of Yoga very much.

A most important point is to *move as slowly in coming out of a Yoga posture as in going into it.* If you do not do this, you will lose much of the benefit. You will be reminded of this frequently throughout the exercise instructions.

Moving slowly also results in a rather profound insight regarding our desperate and often hysterically hurried way of life. We seldom move slowly enough in life. By going through a series of slow movements every day, you will come to realize how far from normal leisure, repose, relaxation and serenity you are while immersed, for the greater part unknowingly, in "the pace that kills." Modern man's customary pace helps destroy his ability to perceive the depth, mystery and beauty of life.

## Easy Does It in Yoga

A rule to keep in mind throughout your practice of Yoga is: THE SLOWER YOU MOVE, THE MORE YOU WILL GET OUT OF THE EXERCISES PHYSICALLY AND MENTALLY.

The second uppermost rule is: HOLD THE POSITION MOTION-LESS. When you have stretched, in slow-motion, into the posture and have reached the point past which you cannot comfortably stretch, you must then hold the posture for the prescribed amount of time *without moving a muscle of your body*. Never fidget, shift around or attempt to adjust your body because you might have the impression that by so doing you can add another half inch or so to your stretch. Once you are in a posture, stretched to your comfortable enjoyable limit, any movements that you make will detract from the physical and mental effects that are taking place at the time. So no matter how you might be tempted to move or adjust your body, hold your posture absolutely motionless and make sure that you are breathing slowly and completely.

Never tug, strain or pull strenuously at any time in Yoga. The rule is to stretch until you feel uncomfortable. Whenever you feel any part of your body to be genuinely uncomfortable, then you know you are applying yourself too strenuously.

All Yoga exercises involve a specific time duration. Most of the stretching postures in this book start at ten seconds. Whether you are moving into a posture, holding it, or coming out of it, you will have to count the time silently to yourself. Count the seconds as follows: "One hundred and one, one hundred and two, one hundred and three," etc. Each count should take approximately one second.

At this point I wish to point out that anyone, regardless of age, who has a history of heart condition, other serious medical condition or has had a severe accident should by all means consult with their physician regarding the practice of Yoga. Show him the Yoga exercises and proceed only according to his advice. It has been my experience, however, throughout the years that an overwhelming majority of doctors not only approve of the practice of Yoga for persons of all ages but urge that practice.

TO SUMMARIZE:

Practice . . .

in a quiet room.
in comfortable, suitable clothing.
at approximately the same time each day.
with correct slow-motion.
holding your positions motionless.
without force or strain.
with a serene attitude.

# PART TWO

# Gentle and Beneficial Yoga Exercises for Every Part of Your Body

# CHAPTER EIGHT

# Beauty and Health
# for the Toes

*About the Toes*

A student of mine, who is an attractive young lady, told me the following story. She had been asked out on a date by a tall, handsome, athletic medical student whom she had liked very much for a long time and with whom she had secretly wished to go out. It was a happy evening for her when he came to pick her up. He suggested that they walk to where they were going, which was a distance of about eight blocks. The young woman was in her early twenties, the young man was about thirty. She found that after the fourth block her feet hurt so much, especially in the region of the big toe, that she was compelled to tell him of this fact and they took a taxi the rest of the way.

Being a medical student he inquired as to what was wrong. She revealed to him that nothing was organically or pathologically wrong with her feet, it turned out to be only a lack of exercise and the wearing of improper shoes that made her unable to walk a normal distance. She told me that it was the most humiliating moment of her life when she saw the expression on his face change from sympathetic interest to a look of incomprehension and poorly concealed disdain upon realizing that she was simply not up to walking more than four blocks. He was a man who believed in leading a vigorous, healthy life. That first date was her last with him.

She was wise enough to take the incident to heart and rather than blaming the young man for being over-critical she blamed herself for having allowed her body to get into such condition that a presumably minor part could so disable her. For most modern people the toes have become excessively tender, nearly vestigial organs. They are the source of tens of millions of dollars of income for chiropodists, orthopedic shoe manufacturers and patent medicine companies. First, we do not use proper shoes. The toes are pinched and not allowed any freedom of movement. Living as we do in cities we do not have enough occasion to walk on grass, on sand or simply barefoot on mother earth. Walking on grass or sand restores the toes to their normal condition.

The strength has been lost from these organs. Also most of the use of them has been lost. The use of the toes may be subtle, but that does not make it less important. The toes are very significant in maintaining our proper sense and condition of balance. Once the sense of balance is impaired, however slightly, your natural poise and grace is diminished, and your normal self-confidence is deteriorated. The toes are made to give the body that "spring" in walking which is so beautiful to see and that "springy" feeling of vitality, well-being and life.

In walking the toes were made to spread at each step and to grip the ground. Nature did not design them to be merely five brute appendages to lie inertly at each step. If you ever have occasion to observe primitive people or people whose way of life enables them to use their toes in a natural normal manner, you will see that the toes in walking are used very much as the fingers would be used if you were walking on all fours.

Loss of strength and improper use now make the toes subject to many ailments. If in your particular case you are fortunately not affected with any overt symptoms of neglect, you may be sure that the ill usage of these small vital parts contributes to the general fatigue that chronically burdens so many millions of people. When one part of the body is abused and fatigued the effect spreads like ink in water. It permeates the entire organism. The most familiar example of this is the eyes. The eyes get tired from too much reading or reading in a bad light. The entire nervous system is consequently affected and the whole body shares in the fatigue. Thus it is important to make sure that *every* part of the body is in proper normal condition.

So we see that the habitual inattention to and neglect of the toes results in diminished strength, danger of common ailments in that area and also loss of normal balance, spring and walking control. The subject of toes may seem minor, trivial and even silly but considering these factors you can see how the old parable about "for want of a nail, the war was lost" applies to it. Let us then go into the first Yoga exercise in this book, an exercise which applies directly to the toes.

## Exercise 1: THE BACKWARD BEND ON THE TOES

STRENGTHENING A NEGLECTED AND ABUSED
AREA.

### *How to practice this exercise*

1. Place your body on a mat on your knees and on your toes as shown in Fig. 1. Sit with the full weight of your body on your heels. Your knees and feet are together. Let your palms rest lightly on your thighs. If you experience discomfort or have difficulty in sitting in this manner then do not go any further in the performing of the posture but make sitting in this position your exercise for the present. That is, sit and adjust your weight slowly onto your heels until you can sit on your heels and toes for 5 full seconds, counting the seconds in the manner previously instructed. When you can accomplish this then proceed with the rest of the exercise as follows.

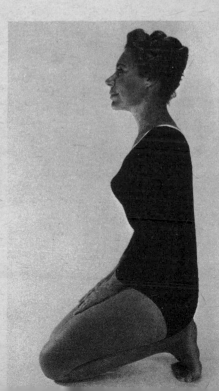

*Figure 1*

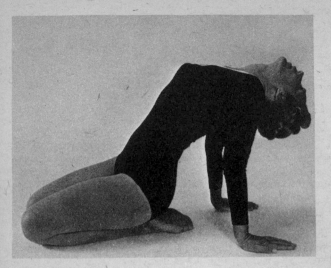

Figure 2

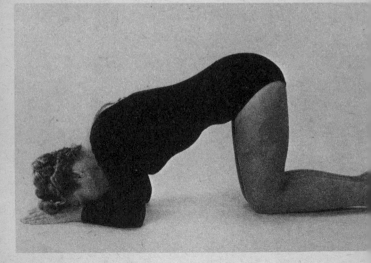

Figure 3

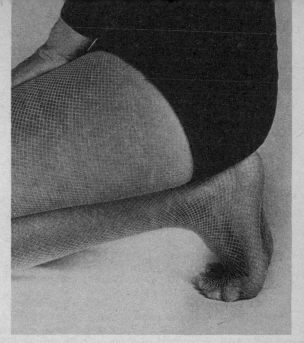

*Figure 4*

2. Place your hands on the floor at your sides. With your fingertips touching the floor, very slowly move your hands backward a few inches at a time until your hands are behind your body, on your palms, at shoulder width, with your fingertips facing to the rear, as shown in Fig. 2. Your arms are now supporting much of the weight of your upper body.

3. Lower your head slowly until it hangs back limply.

4. Hold the position *motionless* for the count of 5.

5. Slowly raise your head. Slowly and carefully walk your hands forward until you are in your beginning position as in Fig. 1.

6. Since you will repeat this technique 3 times, it is advisable to relieve the pressure upon your toes after each time by going all the way forward until you are resting on your elbows and knees with your forehead or cheek resting on the mat. This in itself, is a delightfully relaxing position. (See Fig. 3.)

7. When you have thus rested and relieved your toes for a few moments, simply sit back up on your heels into your original starting position and perform *The Backward Bend on the Toes* over again. (See "close up" in Fig. 4.)

NOTE: It is not only important but it is essential to rest for a few moments after performing any Yoga stretching technique. This makes certain that you experience the full relaxation and relief from tension that the technique brings to all or part of your body. It also prevents you from hurrying, straining and subjecting yourself to exhaustion rather than developing the calmness and endurance that comes from the correct practice of Yoga.

### Benefits to you from toe exercises

1. *The Backward Bend on the Toes* strengthens the toes and restores them to full use and normal health.
2. It stretches and at the same time strengthens the great tendons along the sole of the foot, strengthening and relieving tension in the arch.
3. It provides a highly therapeutic limbering of the knee joints, restoring normal flexibility to the tendons and ligaments in that delicate area.
4. It stretches the tightness and tension out of the great muscles along the top of the thighs. (You can feel this sensation the very first time you practice the technique.)
5. It provides a mild backward stretch to the spinal column, relieving tension throughout the area, adjusting the vertebrae in a gentle manner and helping to restore youthful limberness and elasticity to the spine.
6. It aids in reducing excess weight in the abdomen.
7. It provides a mild but significant increase in circulation in the head, refreshing the organs and glands in the head and face.

*The Backward Bend on the Toes* happens to be one of the more difficult Yoga exercises. It is taught first because the exercises in Part Two of this book are organized to work upon the body from the toes up to the head and are not presented in order of difficulty. Most of the techniques are much easier to master than this particular one.

### Practice schedule

Begin by holding the posture for 5 seconds. Add 2 seconds per week until you are holding it for 20 seconds. Repeat the posture 2 times at each practice period.

### Special hints

If you have difficulty in getting into the posture or in sitting for the required length of time on your heels, it means that your toes are in a weakened, atrophied condition. That is the reason why it is absolutely necessary for you to begin practicing these techniques right now. Leaving your body alone when it is weak and out of condition in certain areas can only result in additional weakening, thus progressing downward from then on. By taking those deteriorated or out of condition spots and areas "in your own hands" by means of Yoga, you can rejuvenate them to a splendid, vibrant condition of health and well-being.

Go only as far as you can in this and any other Yoga posture. Never force yourself to go beyond the limit of comfort. In the short time of a few weeks you will find yourself able to get into *The Backward Bend on the Toes* completely and easily. It is a natural position for the human body to assume and anyone who practices methodically and regularly will be able to get into it. Once you are in it and able to hold it for the prescribed time in the correct way, your body will receive all the benefits listed and you will experience a resurgence of health, physical fitness and the improvement of appearance that comes with these.

Be sure your neck is completely relaxed and limp and that your head hangs back in this posture. Keep your eyes closed while you are holding it motionless.

Remember to come out of this posture as slowly as you can. Coming out of a posture in correct slow motion is as important as going into it slowly. If you "collapse" out of a posture or rush out of it through impatience, you tend to negate much of its benefits.

# CHAPTER NINE

# Beauty and Health
# for the Feet

## About the Feet

We are accustomed to thinking of our feet as some sort of brute organ, like a hoof. We have subsequently come to treat our feet accordingly. The foot is, however, a delicate and sensitive organ which is obliged to perform an enormous load of work for us. Think of it. You will have to walk, run, and stand on your feet for the rest of your life. How can you afford to abuse such a vital part!

We do, however, abuse them. We force them into leather contrivances that constrict them and prevent them from breathing. Women are even worse offenders than men in regard to forcing the feet into shoes that twist them out of their natural shape. On top of this abuse we seldom or never exercise these parts in a way that really does them any good.

One of the main things that is wrong with our feet is that the upper tendons from the toes to the ankle are tightened and stiff through tension and lack of normal use. The foot is thus subject to muscle cramps.

It is a known fact that the feet are one of the main parts of the body to be attacked by painful arthritis. We have had scores upon scores of people come to our classes and tell us after a few weeks that for the first time in years the pain in their feet has diminished. Keeping an area flexible and with proper circulation going through it has much to do with preventing a considerable amount of the danger of arthritis settling in that area. We believe that this especially applies to the feet.

The feet should contain strong muscles, limber, pliable ligaments and tendons, nerves free from tension, and esthetic form equal to any Greek statue. Anyone's feet can be in this condition with proper care.

## Exercise 2: THE JAPANESE SITTING POSITION

STRETCHING TENSION OUT OF THE TOES, FEET
AND ARCH.

### How to practice this exercise

1. Place yourself on your hands and knees on your mat. Make sure your knees and feet are together. Extend your toes outward so that the tops of your arches are lying flat against the floor.

2. Come back into a sitting position so that your buttocks sit upon your heels. Once you are comfortably in this position, your entire body weight should rest upon your heels. Sit erectly.

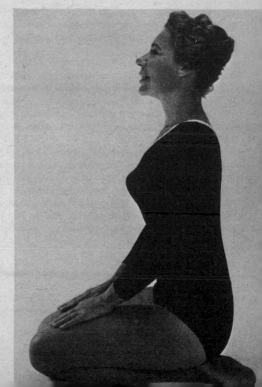

*Figure 5*

3. *The Japanese Sitting Position* is completed when your hands are placed palms down on your thighs as in Fig. 5.

### Benefits to you

*The Backward Bend on the Toes, The Japanese Sitting Position* (the present posture), and the next posture, *The Backward Bend* form a small family of related exercises. The effects upon many parts of the body are the same in each of them, only the emphasis or concentration is different.

1. *The Japanese Sitting Position* stretches the tendons that reach from the top of the toes to the inside of the ankle. You experience a delightful stretching sensation and you can actually feel the tension being relieved from this tight area.

2. The knee joint is limbered.

3. Considerable tension is eliminated from the upper thigh muscle.

4. The ankle itself is stretched in a direction which is of great benefit in removing unnatural tightness that has settled in that area.

### Practice schedule

This is a Yoga technique that has no specific time limit on it. At the beginning, however, you may find that your ankles and feet are particularly stiff and out of condition and that the time you can sit in the position will be limited.

Once you can sit in this posture without undue discomfort, you should begin substituting it whenever possible for your customary chair sitting position. Chair sitting in itself is not healthful for certain parts of the body. Since you are going to spend a certain amount of your time sitting anyway, you may as well use that time to bring about the wonderful results to your muscles, tendons, and nerves that come from sitting in this manner.

So when you sit down to read or watch television or relax with a hobby, it is best to use this position as long as you comfortably can in place of the old slumping-in-a-chair sitting habit. As time goes by your body will adapt more and more to this posture and you will find that you will be able to sit for greater lengths of time and eventually it will become quite normal and natural for you. At that point the parts of your body affected will undergo a profound regeneration.

### Special hints

If you have difficulty getting into the position go only as far as you can and hold your farthest position for the count of 5. Then, add 5 seconds each week to the time that you hold the position as far as you can get into it. You will find that in a very short while you will have worked your

way into the complete *Japanese Sitting Position* and all the benefits that
come from it will be taking place.

For prolonged sitting, you may employ the variation of allowing your
heels to separate slightly so long as your big toes are together.

## Exercise 3: THE BACKWARD BEND

STRETCHING TENSION OUT OF THE FEET AND
ANKLES.

*How to practice this exercise*

1. Place your body in *The Japanese Sitting Position* which you have
just learned in the previous exercise (Fig. 6).
2. Place your fingertips on the floor at your sides (Fig. 7).

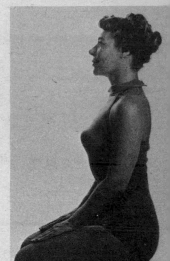

*Figure 7*

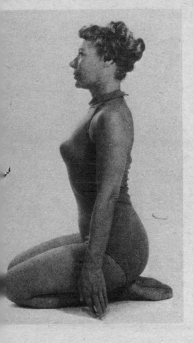

*Figure 6*

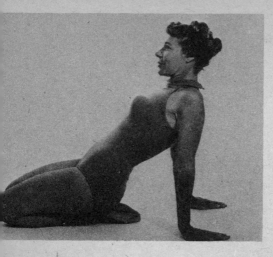

Figure 8

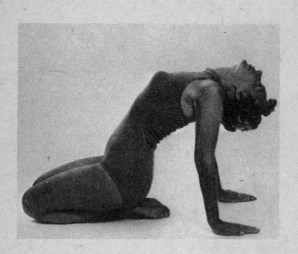

Figure 9

3. Walk slowly back with your fingers a few inches at a time until your hands are from one to two feet behind your feet, palms down, at approximately shoulder width, with your elbows straight and your fingers pointing in the same direction as your toes (Fig. 8).

4. Let your head drop slowly back until it is hanging down with your neck completely limp and relaxed.

5. Without removing your buttocks from your heels and without taking any of the weight of your body off your feet, push your abdomen upward and forward thus arching your spine in a backward direction (Fig. 9).

6. With your eyes closed and breathing regularly, hold this position for 10 seconds. Count the time to yourself as instructed, saying, one hundred and one, one hundred and two, etc.

7. Relieve the stretch of your spine and lower your abdomen to its original relaxed position. Raise your head slowly.

8. Walk slowly forward with your hands until you are sitting upright in *The Japanese Sitting Position* once again with your hands palms down on your thighs.

9. Come forward onto your elbows with your forehead or cheek resting upon the mat, thus relieving the pressure from your feet.

### Benefits to you

1. *The Backward Bend* provides a stretching, limbering and working out of the toes, feet and ankles, removing tension from these areas and restoring their strength and normal use.

2. There is a therapeutic stretching of the spine in a backward direction.

3. It develops the rib cage, chest and bust.

4. This posture is very good for improving the posture and even for overcoming minor postural difficulties.

5. Blood circulation in the head is mildly stimulated.

6. Deep relaxation is achieved and you will experience an immediate relief from overall body tension.

7. Tension is stretched out of the spine, abdominal muscles and the front of the thighs.

8. There is a surge of renewed energy after performing this posture.

### Practice schedule

Repeat *The Backward Bend* 3 times.

Hold your farthest position for 10 seconds during the first week.

Add 5 seconds to your holding time every week until you are holding it for 30 seconds.

### Special hints

To repeat this posture the second and third time, you simply raise your body from the position in which you are relieving the pressure from your feet and sit slowly and smoothly back into *The Japanese Sitting Position*.

Keep your eyes closed throughout the holding of the posture. This will greatly help you in experiencing its tremendous relaxing effect.

Remember to move always in slow motion. When you are holding the posture and counting the seconds to yourself, do not move at all: Be as motionless as a statue.

Breathe through your nose throughout the posture.

## Exercise 4: THE SIMPLE POSTURE

A MORE NATURAL SITTING POSITION AND A
PREPARATORY POSTURE FOR THE HALF LOTUS.

### How to practice this exercise

Very little instruction is needed for this technique since in the

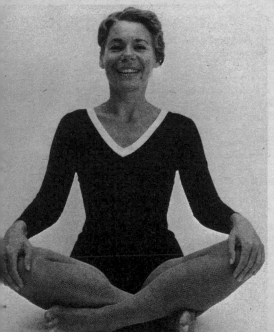

*Figure 10*

study of Yoga its function is very much a preparation for *The Half Lotus* sitting position which is taught next.

Simply sit on your mat in the cross-legged posture as shown in Fig. 10.

### Benefits to you

1. This posture, simple as it is, is infinitely superior for the circulation throughout the legs than the chair sitting position.
2. It begins to loosen the ankle, knee and hip joints.
3. It is calming for the nerves and mind.

### Practice schedule

You should sit in this *Simple Posture* whenever you can during the day or evening. Substitute it at all possible occasions for your usual chair sitting position. You can employ *The Simple Posture* while reading, watching television, or while sitting to rest. If your family has a positive attitude toward your study of Yoga you would do well to draw your legs up in this fashion even when you sit on a chair such as during mealtime.

Use this as your regular sitting position until such time that your legs are limber enough to use *The Half Lotus* in its place.

## Exercise 5: THE HALF LOTUS

LIMBERS THE ANKLES.

### How to practice this exercise

1. Sit on your mat with your legs extended straight out in front of you, heels and toes together.
2. Bend your left leg at the knee and bring your foot up toward your body so that you can grasp your left foot with your hands. Your left knee is against or near the mat rather than in the air.
3. Place the sole of your left foot against the inside of your right thigh. Do not allow this foot to slide underneath your right thigh. Draw your left heel up as closely as you can to your groin (Fig. 11).
4. Now bend your right leg at the knee so that you can grasp your right foot with your hands. Your right knee is toward or against the mat.
5. Lift your right foot up with your hands and place the outside blade of your right foot on the cleft where your left thigh and calf come together. Be sure to draw your right heel as close to your groin as comfort permits. The sole of your right foot should tend to face upward.
6. Rest your wrists on your knees as depicted in Fig. 12.

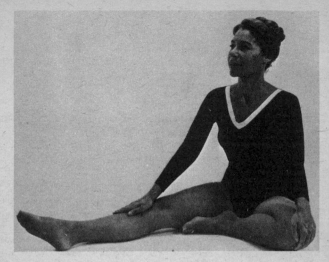

*Figure 11*

*Figure 12*

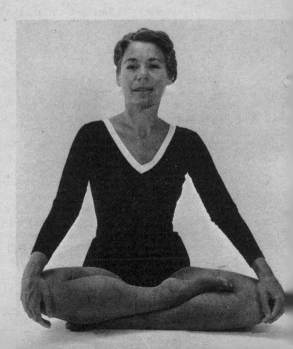

### Benefits to you

1. The benefit of this ancient and wonderful sitting posture to your feet is that it loosens and limbers the ankles, removing stiffness and tension in that area.

2. The same effects occur to the knee and hip joints, which have become stiff through years of improper use and lack of correct exercise.

3. Circulation in the region of the ankle, knee, and hip joints is improved. A number of my students have informed me that arthritic pain in the feet, knee, and hip joints has been relieved by their practice of *The Half Lotus*.

4. This sitting posture has a wonderful effect upon certain little used and seldom reached tendons, ligaments, and muscles. The great tendons that run along the inside of the thighs from the knee to the groin, tendons which are never worked out in the course of our usual daily physical activity, are stretched, rejuvenated, and strengthened by *The Half Lotus*. Much accumulated tension in that particular area is relieved. The small tendons and the tissues of the groin and of the pelvic area are stretched and worked out.

5. Once you have stretched your way into this posture and your body has become accustomed to it, then you will experience genuine sitting comfort for perhaps the first time. In this sittting position, a condition of physical balance and calmness is achieved. Fidgeting becomes unnecessary and sitting is no longer subject to periodic agitation as it is, for the greater part unknowingly, in our Western chair sitting position.

6. This is the most comfortable sitting position for the practice of meditation. One of the objectives of Yogic meditation is the resting of the fretful mind. Meditation itself will be taught in some detail in a later portion of this book.

7. The banishing of tension from the legs in *The Half Lotus* results in a relaxing effect upon the entire nervous system.

8. The posture tends to slow metabolism and breathing. The breathing becomes longer and less erratic. This in turn has an enormous influence upon quieting and calming the mind.

### Practice schedule

There is no formal time limit on the holding of *The Half Lotus*. You should sit in the posture until you no longer feel comfortable. When this point is reached you should then reverse the position of your legs.

It is important to come out of this posture correctly or else you will feel a strain and discomfort. The way to do it is to very slowly lift your right foot off your left leg and place it on the floor. Then, slowly, with the aid of your hands, straighten your leg out until it is in front of you once again. You may softly and slowly massage your knee at this point. Do not massage it vigorously. Then straighten your left leg out and do the same thing.

When you are ready, bend your right leg, placing the sole of your right foot against the inside of your left thigh and then bend your left leg, placing the outside blade of that foot on the cleft between the right thigh and calf. Thus you will be sitting in *The Half Lotus* position with your legs reversed.

As soon as you are able, perform all your breathing exercises in this position.

### Special hints

*The Half Lotus* is a natural sitting position for human beings. Chair sitting as we practice it nearly universally in the West is, on the other hand, an unnatural body position. Sitting in a chair is in reality less comfortable than sitting in one of the Yoga cross-legged positions. This may seem untrue in the light of whatever initial discomfort or stiffness you may experience in the very beginning. Whatever discomfort you experience with the Yoga sitting positions is simply the result of wrong lifelong sitting habits plus the fact that the joints of your legs have become unnaturally stiff and inflexible from lack of proper use. Once your body, through pleasant regular practice, becomes accustomed to *The Half Lotus,* you will experience what I mean when I refer to genuine comfort. You will be able to look back and realize the unnaturalness of chair sitting and its negative effect upon the health. Once you are comfortable in *The Half Lotus* you can sit in it indefinitely without feeling uncomfortable, fidgety or restless; but, let's see you sit in a chair without moving for even a moderate period of time. It becomes literally a form of torture. Take note of people sitting in chairs. They are compelled to move their bodies, adjust their position, shift around, fidget, or cross their legs every few minutes. This is because chair sitting presses the backs of the thighs and the buttocks in such a manner that the nerves are irritated. At the same time the position of the legs, hanging down as they do, makes proper circulation more difficult.

I am frequently asked, "How should I hold my back when I am sitting in *The Half Lotus,* or in *The Simple Posture?* Should I keep my back ramrod straight?" The answer is that a ramrod, rigid spine is an extreme posture for the body to be in and is not necessarily synonymous with an "erect" spine. The best rule for keeping your spine erect, is as follows: Keep your ears above your shoulders and keep your nose on a line above your navel. When sitting in *The Half Lotus* with your body held as this little rule describes, your spine will be correctly straight. You will find that there is much leeway for relaxation of the shoulders and back muscles.

It is advisable not to slump while sitting in any of the Yoga sitting postures.

A point of uppermost importance is that in the case of most beginning students the knee of the top leg in *The Half Lotus* posture will not lie down flat toward the mat in a relaxed manner, but will rather stand up in the air due to the stiffness of the ankle and tendons of the leg. You must never under any circumstances manipulate this upraised knee with your hand. Never work it up and down, no matter how gently. Never push it or lean on it. Nor should you even expend muscular effort with that leg itself in order to help lower it further. By working or manipulating the upraised knee in any manner you are placing yourself in danger of straining a joint or pulling a muscle or tendon. Here is a notable instance of effort being a detriment in Yoga. The weight alone of that leg will in time gently and slowly stretch out those ligaments, tendons and muscles which are making the hip, knee, and especially the ankle joint stiff and unyielding. This is the only way that the leg should lower itself to the completed position. It is the only natural, safe way that will result in natural limberness and long lasting benefits.

# CHAPTER TEN

# Beauty and Health
# for the Legs

## *About the Legs*

Here we are on familiar ground. I cannot count the innumerable times that women students of mine have asked me what they can do to improve the appearance of their legs. Not only are legs a major factor in the beauty of a woman, but, constituting such an enormous part of the human body, they are a major factor in the general health and physical fitness of both men and women. Let us look then at the ideas of beauty regarding women's legs.

It is strange how, like styles of clothing, ideas of beauty regarding women's shapes and legs vary in time and place. Way back when the hour glass figure was considered to be the quintessence of beauty and attractiveness, the legs of those women must have corresponded with that hefty form. During the pre-World War I era a rather emaciated and woefully out of condition figure and legs were thought to be the height of loveliness. In the nineteen twenties the style of the flapper took over with her hardy trim athletic limbs. Regardless of the esthetics of that style there were at least some overtones of vigor and health to those Charleston dancers. Then came Betty Grable and her frank, uninhibitedly full-legged pulchritude which verged ever so slightly and ever so subtly on the flesh and which was tremendously feminine and enormously attractive to men.

At present we are in an era where for some reason countless millions upon millions of dollars are spent on propagating the notion that thin legs as such are looked upon as universally beautiful or simply desirable and attractive to men.

The question is: Are you to be forever subject to this fluctuation of style and taste? Are you to have to go through the harrowing process of reshaping your body to suit whatever current style is declared to be beautiful?

Is there not, rather, a range of qualities and characteristics (measurements, if you prefer) within which any woman's legs are considered to be beautiful?

Yoga would maintain that though there is no one exact universal measurement standard for feminine beauty that applies to a woman's entire shape or any part thereof, there is, however, a simple general standard which can enable a woman to be confident that her particular natural beauty in any area is developed and being revealed to its utmost. This is a standard of health and proper conditioning. Applied specifically to the legs it would consist of the following qualities.

1. A smooth, good complexion in the skin of the legs.
2. The legs should be free from unsightly protruding veins and from flabbiness.
3. The legs should be firm enough to reflect a healthy state and proper muscle tone.
4. The legs should be correctly proportioned to the individual woman's height, normal weight and body type.

Objective tests have proven the fallacy of thinking that slimness of the total figure or of the legs alone *for its own sake* is what men actually prefer. The rather brutal truth of these surveys was that while a minority of men enjoy being seen in public with women whose forms are fashion model thin, that is as far as it goes along any avenue of real or meaningful human relationship. The overwhelming majority of men indicated a strong preference and attraction to a full, vibrant and healthy-looking figure in a woman.

A woman must not reduce her legs merely for the sake of having slender legs. She must rather reduce her legs, if necessary, only so that they harmonize with her general shape when her body as a whole is in a normal condition of health and fitness.

Here is the greatness and practicality of Yoga. It slowly develops and adjusts the entire body to its most harmonious proportions. Weight is lost and slimness is achieved according to the natural inherent beauty lying dormant within you.

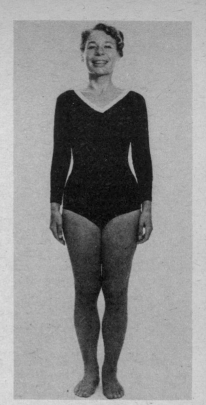

*Figure 13*

### Exercise 6: THE STANDING TWIST

WORKING OUT EVERY MUSCLE IN A TWISTING
MANNER.

#### How to practice this exercise

1. Stand erectly with your abdomen pulled in and your chest out
and held high. Stand as tall as you can as if you are being suspended in
place by a cord attached to the top of your head. Keep your heels together
and your toes slightly apart (Fig. 13).

2. With your arms straight and your elbows locked, raise your arms
slowly up in front of you until they are extended straight out at approximately eye level with the thumbs of each hand touching each other. As
you raise your arms slowly from your sides you should inhale one long

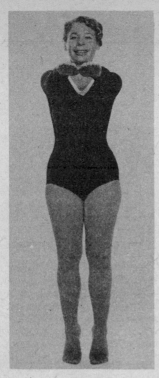
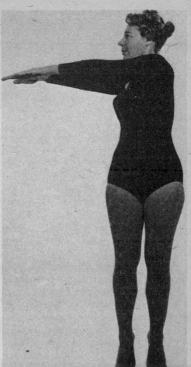

*Figure 14*                              *Figure 15*

complete breath. When your arms are up in front of you, commence breathing in a normal manner.

3. This step is to be performed at the same time as step number 2. As you raise your arms forward, rise slowly up on your toes (Fig. 14).

4. Now begin moving your arms, hands touching always, toward your right. Your toes are facing forward while your hands and arms are turning, in slow motion, toward your right. This movement creates a twisting throughout your body in a corkscrew manner from your ankles up through your pelvis, waist and spine.

Keep your eyes focused on your fingertips during this movement and while holding the posture. Move your hands and arms as far around to your right as you can without discomfort or undue strain.

5. When you have reached your farthest position toward your right (which should place your arms at approximately a 90 degree angle to your feet), hold this position for 10 seconds without moving (Fig. 15).

6. Bring your arms slowly back to their original position facing forward.

7. Very slowly lower your arms back to your sides as you come down from your tiptoe position and stand flatfooted again.

8. Repeat the exact same procedure but the next time move your arms around to your left side.

9. When you are finished moving around to the left, holding the posture for the prescribed time, and returning to your normal standing position, you have performed *The Standing Twist* once. The complete movement consists of one twist on each side.

## Benefits to you

1. The muscles and connective tissues of the legs are stretched in a spiral manner which strengthens the legs, tones the muscles and aids in slimming excess adipose tissue from them.

2. *The Standing Twist* helps reduce the waist and makes that region more supple and flexible.

3. The spine is twisted in a spiral manner and its normal flexibility is restored. Stiffness and tension are removed from the muscles, ligaments and tendons around the spinal column. It is at the same time a wholesome gentle stretch for the nerves that emanate from the spinal column, and highly therapeutic for the entire nervous system.

4. Tension is removed from the neck.

5. This posture greatly aids in restoring your natural sense of balance. In addition there is an increase of the poise and grace that is always lost when the sense of balance is decreased through lack of proper bodily use.

## Practice schedule

Do *The Standing Twist* 3 times on each side, alternating from left to right.

Begin by holding your farthest position for 10 seconds.

Add 5 seconds each week until you are holding the posture for 30 seconds.

## Special hints

The development or restoration of your sense of balance is an important effect of this exercise. You will invariably lose your balance from time to time in the beginning and you will come abruptly down from your tiptoe position and have to regain your balance momentarily by standing flatfooted. When wobbling or total loss of balance occurs, it is very important for you not to react to it. Don't laugh, giggle or manifest disappointment, even to the mere saying of "shucks" to yourself. It is important to pretend that nothing at all has happened. It is the same as if you were learning how to play the piano. Naturally, you would strike wrong notes with more frequency during the beginning stages. If you were to stop and react with a laugh or an expression of disappointment every time you did this, you would not only slow down your progress in learning to play the piano but you would be continually "throwing yourself off" your concentration on the exercise you are attempting to perform. It is the same with Yoga. Though Yoga is fun one must practice it as a kind of dignified, calm and controlled fun so that you do not break your concentration and hinder your progress in it.

The keeping of your eyes on your fingertips throughout the exercise not only plays an important part in making sure that you are performing the posture correctly but in itself it helps promote and develop the faculty of mental concentration.

It is important to note that the higher up you rise on your toes the easier it will be to keep your balance throughout the exercise. While it may seem like a contradiction, by rising as high as you can on your toes you will come to be standing on a sort of level pad extending from the tips of your toes to the ball of your foot. This "little platform" is a great aid in keeping yourself balanced throughout the exercise. If you do not rise this high on your toes but merely lift your heels a short distance off the floor instead, your balance depends on the continual adjustment of your calf muscles and you have much more of a tendency to waver, wobble and eventually lose your balance.

You will note a remarkable effect upon your stance and walk when you become proficient in *The Standing Twist*. A new grace and confidence of bearing develops and in time will last long after you have finished your workout period.

As with all Yoga techniques, keep a serene demeanor and attitude while practicing. Breathe calmly and remind yourself to be relaxed throughout the posture. Serenity comes to be a habit and eventually a characteristic trait. People sense both the calm that Yoga gives its students and also the control or discipline that the student comes to have over her body and mind. Students never cease coming to me and reporting how some person who has known them for years has suddenly remarked upon their relaxation, calmness and self assurance and asked them what accounted for it.

If for some reason you are not able to perform *The Standing Twist* on your toes, then you should begin, for the first two weeks, to do this exercise without rising on your toes. Simply do the same movements but stand flatfooted throughout. I urge you, however, to attempt to rise up on your toes as soon as you can.

### Exercise 7: THE ALTERNATE LEG PULL

TENSION IS REMOVED AND FLEXIBILITY AND
LIMBERNESS ARE REGAINED THROUGHOUT THE
ENTIRE LEG.

*How to practice this exercise*

1. Sit on your mat with your legs extended straight out in front
of you, toes and heels together and palms resting lightly on your thighs.

2. Bend your left leg at the knee and bring your left foot toward
your body so you can grasp it with your hands.

3. With the aid of your hands place the sole of your left foot against
(not under) the inside of your right thigh. Draw your left heel as closely
as you can without discomfort toward your groin (Fig. 16).

4. Keeping your back straight and your chest high, raise both your
hands straight out in front of you until they are in the air slightly above
eye level (Fig. 17).

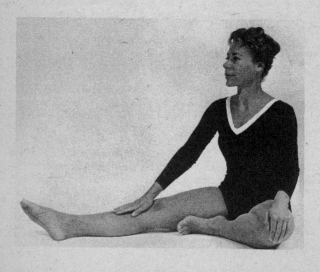

*Figure 16*

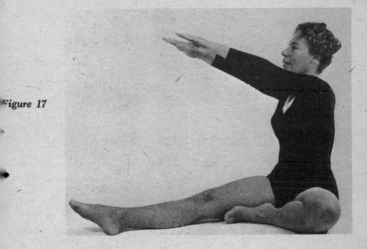

Figure 17

5. In slow motion bend forward at your waist and attempt to grasp with your hands the farthest part of your extended right leg that you can reach. You should take at least 10 full seconds to perform this forward moving slow-motion stretch.

Take a firm grip on that part which will be either your foot, ankle, calf, knee, or thigh depending upon how stiff you have become (Fig. 18).

6. Having your grip, now bend your elbows outward slowly and gently (Fig. 19) so that you pull yourself down until you cannot comfortably stretch any further. Never strain, tug or pull strenuously in any Yoga stretch. It is not necessary and will actually retard your progress. Let your head hang limply toward your right knee. Your ultimate goal in this posture is to be able to rest your forehead against the knee of your extended leg as in Fig. 20.

7. Now that you have your stretch, hold it absolutely motionless for 10 seconds. Count the time to yourself in the prescribed manner. DO NOT MOVE, FIDGET, ADJUST YOURSELF, OR PULL BACKWARD OR FORWARD WITH THE IDEA OF GAINING AN EXTRA FRACTION OF AN INCH IN YOUR STRETCH. Such movements will detract from the results.

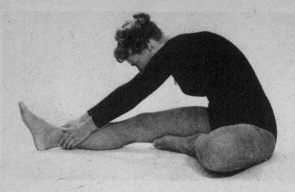

Figure 18

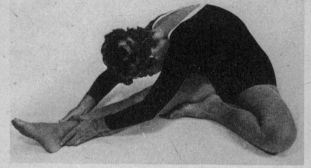

Figure 19

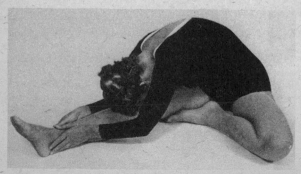

Figure 20

8. When you have finished your stretch, slowly, bows, release your grip upon your extended leg, and, sli up the front of your leg, slowly straighten up out of the postu sure that your head is the last part of your body to straighten up.

9. Straighten your left leg out to your original beginning position.

10. Bend your right leg at the knee so you can grasp your right foot with your hand and repeat the exact same exercise on the other side, stretching your left leg and the right side of your back.

## Benefits to you

1. *The Alternate Leg Pull* stretches, strengthens and tones every ligament, tendon and muscle of the leg.

2. It slims and reshapes the legs.

3. It restores youthful flexibility to the legs, giving them new life, strength and endurance.

4. It removes tension from every place in which it is deeply hidden throughout the legs (especially the back of the legs from the heel to the buttocks), buttocks, back and spine.

5. It stretches, limbers and tones the muscles of the back, making the back youthfully flexible and supple.

6. The normal elasticity of the spinal column itself is restored.

7. Flabbiness in the waist, thighs and abdomen is removed.

8. The muscles of the shoulders, arms, and upper back are strengthened.

## Practice schedule

Perform *The Alternate Leg Pull* as instructed 3 times on each side, alternating from one leg to the other.

Begin by holding the posture for 10 seconds.

After the first week add 5 seconds to your holding time each week until you are holding the posture for 45 seconds. (At this point you will have attained tremendous elasticity and limberness.)

## Special hints

*The Alternate Leg Pull* is one of the fastest working of all the major Yoga postures. Its results are gained very quickly and you will be amazed at how soon your head will be approaching your knee as your body begins to "give." You will experience the thrill of regaining your natural condition of youthful flexibility.

Do not bend the knee of your outstretched leg under any circumstances. You may be tempted to bend it a little in order to gain an extra inch or so in your stretch but I assure you that in doing so you will be

will only be cheating yourself out of

slowly while performing this or any other
otherwise. By so doing you are helping
that comes with the correct practice of these

take at least 10 seconds in going into the stretch
out of the stretch. Never come back out of one of
these than you went into it because this virtually erases
a consider tion of its physical and mental results.

When you are stretching your left leg in *The Alternate Leg Pull*, you
will at the same time be stretching the right side of your back. And when
you are stretching your right leg you will be stretching the left side of
your back. This is a complete workout of the entire back of your body
from heels to neck.

The ultimate position of this posture is when your forehead can
rest upon your outstretched knee and your elbows can touch the floor
on either side of that leg. The reaching of your forehead to your knee
will come in a moderately short time and it is a great thrill and feeling
of accomplishment when it happens. It takes a little longer for the elbows
to reach the floor.

Keep your eyes closed throughout the posture and attempt to empty
your mind of extraneous thoughts that might tend to drag you back into
the agitation of the usual daily thinking process. This is a time for resting
the mind as well as for developing the body.

### Exercise 8: THE FULL LOTUS

COMPLETE LIMBERING OF THE ANKLE, KNEE
AND HIP JOINTS.

#### How to practice this exercise

1. Sit on your mat with your legs extended straight out in front of
you.

2. Bend your left leg at the knee, keeping your knee toward the mat,
and bring your left foot toward your body so that you can grasp it with
your hands.

3. Always moving gently and carefully, lift your left foot with
your hands and place it on the top of your right thigh. Draw your left
heel as close to your abdominal wall as you can. If possible your left heel
should be lightly touching your abdomen. Your left foot will tend to rest
on your left thigh with the sole upward (Fig. 21).

4. Now bend your right leg in the same manner so you can grasp
your right foot with both hands.

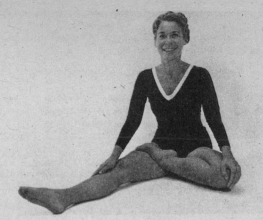

Figure 21

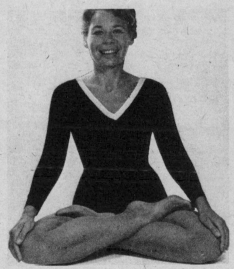

Figure 22

5. Gently and carefully lift your right foot with your hands and place it on top of your left thigh. Draw your right heel as close as you can toward your abdominal wall. In the completed posture, the right heel will also press lightly against your abdominal wall.

6. Rest your wrists or palms lightly on your knees and sit with your back erect (Fig. 22).

63

### Benefits to you

1. *The Full Lotus* posture promotes and restores the natural elasticity of your ankle, knee and hip joints.

2. The tendons and ligaments that run along the inside of your thighs from your knees to your groin are stretched and developed. Deep tension is relieved and new life is restored to these vital tissues.

3. Small seldom-used muscles of the groin are stretched and strengthened.

4. General fatigue, especially fatigue in the legs, is overcome.

5. When sitting in *The Full Lotus* a person's breathing tends to become slower and deeper, which is highly beneficial for the lungs and for the nervous system.

6. *The Full Lotus* helps calm the metabolism.

7. This is a splendid sitting position for the practice of meditation. It is in fact the classic sitting position for the practice of meditation as exemplified by the most ancient statues, pictures and texts of the Orient. Meditation, or the mental exercises for obtaining peace of mind and serenity in the midst of life, will be presented in detail in the section on *Beauty and Health Through Peace of Mind*.

8. Due to the relaxing and calming effect of this sitting posture upon the metabolism and nervous system, the mind tends to become quieted and calm, and you will appear royally serene.

### Practice schedule

As with *The Simple Posture* and *The Half Lotus*, *The Full Lotus* can be employed for as long as you can sit in it without strain or discomfort.

In this case, however, you should pay very careful attention to special hints that follow.

### Special hints

*The Full Lotus* is actually an advanced posture. It is not necessary to master or even use it for the attainment of the physical and mental results that are yours from the practice of Yoga. Be very careful in working your way into this posture. Some people have retained a natural flexibility of the joints of the legs and can slip into *The Full Lotus* quite easily. If you are not one of these fortunate few, however, you will have to work your way slowly and patiently into this posture. Slowness and patience cannot be overemphasized here.

Do not even attempt *The Full Lotus* until you can sit in *The Half Lotus*—and alternate your legs in *The Half Lotus*—*comfortably* for at least 15 minutes.

When you find you have reached the point where you can begin attempting to place your legs in *The Full Lotus* position, never force or pull even with the smallest extra effort in order to get into it.

When you can place your legs into this position, you should sit in *The Full Lotus* for only 3 seconds at a time during the first week. Then add no more than 5 seconds each week to your holding time until you are absolutely certain your legs have adapted to the position.

Be just as methodical in coming out of the posture as in going into it. When helping your legs out of this posture, do so very slowly, a few inches at a time and allow your legs to rest at each stage. Never unfold your legs from *The Full Lotus* and quickly straighten them out in front of you.

Gently and slowly massage your knee joints when coming out of this posture.

# CHAPTER ELEVEN

# Beauty and Health
for the Thighs

## About the Thighs

The thighs are a major danger point regarding feminine beauty because at a certain age they can suddenly begin deteriorating in condition and appearance at a rapid rate. Weight in the thighs is difficult to remove. How many women today are burdened by the extreme means that they find necessary to employ in order to keep their thighs in normal condition? Extreme means range from strenuous exercise courses and massage therapy to unnatural crash diets and even fasting. These methods can get rid of weight in that specific area but the results never last long. Yoga works slower in restoring the healthful condition and beauty of the thighs but the results of Yoga are very long lasting.

## How Yoga Works on the Thighs

The reason is that Yoga works on removing the causes of deterioration in the condition and appearance of the thighs, while most other forms of physical culture or therapy work on removing only the outward symptoms. The problem that many women have with their thighs is in itself one of the best examples of the fallacy of attacking the symptoms of a physical imperfection rather than the cause.

Take for example the way that massage can reduce weight in the thighs. Now a massage is a splendid thing. It is healthful, helpful, relaxing and in many cases can reduce weight. However, when you rub away excess weight in the thighs you may as well be reconciled to the fact that you are going to have to keep on going to the masseur at regular, frequent intervals and, in the course of time, at considerable expense. Nearly as quickly as weight is rubbed away it returns. The same with fasting. Fasting is a marvelous form of general therapy for human beings to engage in provided, of course, that they do so under professional supervision or with complete knowledge of the proper method. A woman can fast for a day or two and stand in front of a mirror and very likely exclaim, "How wonderful, look how sleek and trim my thighs have become and it's so difficult to do anything with them." But wait another week and there it is back again, the same old problem, or rather the same old symptom of your problem manifesting itself in that particular area.

The problem of excessive weight in a certain area of your body is not really a problem of that area. It is a general bodily problem. We see how certain Yoga exercises tend to concentrate their powers upon one particular body area. There is no doubt that some specific exercise can have a greater effect upon one part of the body than another. In the case of the following three exercises their effects are more specifically concentrated on the thighs; stretching, working out and firming them. At the same time the practice of Yoga, even the mere few minutes required every day, has a deeper effect. The Yoga techniques reach deep into the body and affect the glands, stimulating and regenerating them, helping to normalize their functions through the actual physical massage they receive from certain movements and postures and from the improvement in blood circulation through them.

## Effect of Yoga on Glands

The weight of the body is determined to a very great extent by the functioning of the *thyroid gland.* Many Yoga stretching exercises, especially *The Shoulder Stand* and *The Plough,* have a direct effect on this gland. They normalize the activity of the thyroid. Thus one of the end results of your daily practice of a full Yoga exercise routine is to normalize your body weight in general.

Combined with the emphasis that the various exercises place upon special areas of your body, you now have an enormously effective weapon that you can use to overcome any particular figure problem.

By normalizing the function of vital internal glands and organs Yoga enables the body as a whole to slowly but surely undergo a general transformation from its present condition due to the debilitating influences of modern civilization. You can regain normal weight, shape, resiliency, vigor and firmness.

If you are a person who cares about your health and appearance, you can now be free from the eternally recurring torture of crash diets, pills, spartan exercise regimes, expensive therapy and the frustration that comes from removing the outward symptoms of your problem only to see them quickly recur again time after time.

## Exercise 9: THE KNEE AND THIGH STRETCH

FLEXIBILITY RESTORED AND TENSION REMOVED
ALONG THE INSIDES OF THE THIGHS.

### How to practice this exercise

1. Sit on your mat with your legs stretched out in front of you, knees straight, toes and heels together.

2. Bend both legs at the knees and bring your feet toward you, heels together, until the soles of your feet are together as close to your groin as comfort permits.

3. Intertwine your fingers and clasp your hands around both feet (Fig. 23). Sit up erectly throughout this posture.

4. Sitting erectly and holding your feet with your hands, press slowly down as far as you can toward the floor with your knees (Fig. 24).

5. Hold this position motionless for 10 seconds. Close your eyes and count the time slowly to yourself.

6. Slowly and gently relieve the pressure from your legs allowing your knees to rise to their relaxed beginning position (Fig. 23).

7. Remain in this position with your hands clasped on your feet and your back erect, until you are ready to repeat the exercise.

### Benefits to you

1. *The Knee and Thigh Stretch* removes tension from the thighs.

2. It stretches the great and seldom exercised muscles and tendons of the inner thighs restoring their normal, useful flexibility and limberness.

3. It aids in trimming weight from the thighs.

4. It reduces fatigue in the legs due to the releasing of tension that has been trapped in the seldom used areas there. You will experience a resurgence of strength, endurance and new life in your legs and you will be able to walk and stand for greater lengths of time without fatigue.

5. This exercise provides increased bounce and youthful vigor to your walk.

### Practice schedule

During the first week hold *The Knee and Thigh Stretch* for 10 seconds.

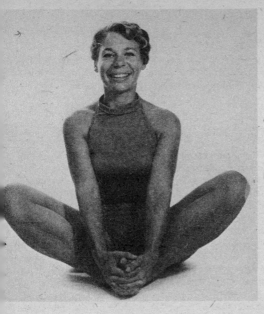

Figure 23

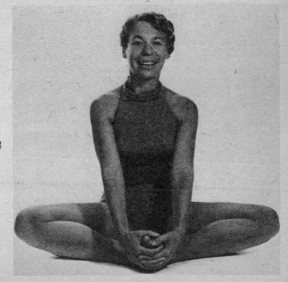

Figure 24

Repeat the exercise 3 times at each sitting.

Add 5 seconds each week to your holding time until you are holding *The Knee and Thigh Stretch* for 30 seconds. If you particularly favor this exercise you may feel free to continually increase your holding time in it providing you do so in a methodical, scientific manner.

### Special hints

The ultimate goal is for the knees to go all the way down to the mat as in Fig. 24. In the beginning most people find that their knees are quite high in the air and that when a few weeks of practice have gone by they do not feel as if they have progressed very much toward the goal. It is a peculiarity of this posture that the progress does not occur in a noticeable straight line. There seems to be no progress at first but suddenly one day the legs just "give" and, as easily as if it has always been natural to you, your knees lower themselves many inches if not all the way. It is a delightful, even thrilling, experience. Remember, these postures *always* work, if you will simply practice them every day.

It is important for you to realize that although you cannot place your body in the ultimate position of the stretching exercises, that does not mean that you are receiving any less results than if you were able to go "all the way." The results of Yoga happen from the very beginning, starting with the first stretch you perform. These results are not dependent upon your being able to go "all the way" into a posture. It is the stretching itself that counts and which brings many invaluable results at every stage along the way.

*Do not slump in this posture.* A good tip to prevent losing the erect position of your back is to allow your head to fall limply backwards so that you are facing up.

*Never bob your knees up and down in an attempt to increase your stretch.* Any such movement will hinder your progress. Remain absolutely motionless throughout. Simply maintain a steady downward pressure upon your legs.

### Exercise 10: THE FOREHEAD TO HEELS STRETCH

TENSION STRETCHED OUT OF THE BACK AND
THIGHS.

#### How to practice this exercise

1. Sit on your mat with your legs extended straight out in front of you with your toes and heels together and your spine erect.
2. Bend your legs at the knees and bring them toward you until the soles of your feet are pressed together and are at approximately the

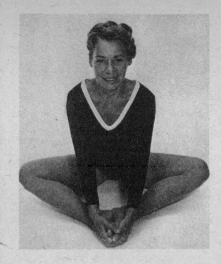

Figure 25

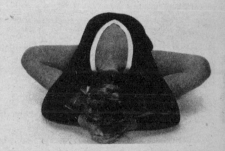

Figure 26

same distance from your body that your knees were when your legs were extended.

3. Intertwine your fingers and clasp your hands over your feet (Fig. 25).

4. Bending your elbows outward, slowly bend forward aiming your forehead for your heels. Aid your stretch by a gentle upward pulling of your feet with your arms. Go down only as far as you can comfortably. Take at least 10 seconds to reach the farthest point of your stretch.

5. When you feel that the slightest amount more of a stretch would be uncomfortable, hold your position motionless for 10 seconds. Fig. 26 shows the complete position, forehead on heels and elbows on the floor.

71

6. At the end of your holding time allow your arms to slowly straighten and let your back straighten up in slow motion with your head being the last part to be raised to an erect position. Take at least 10 seconds to come back up out of your stretch.

7. Remain in this position with your eyes closed and rest for a few minutes. Then repeat *The Forehead to Heels Stretch*.

### Benefits to you

1. Deep tension is removed from the thighs and back.
2. Great elasticity is developed in the thigh muscles and tendons.
3. *The Forehead to Heels Stretch* tones and firms the thigh muscles and aids in reducing weight in that area.
4. The exercise is marvelous for the hip joint. I have been told by many students that chronic pain in the hip joints has disappeared when they practiced this technique.
5. The sacroiliac region of the spine is limbered and adjusted.
6. The entire back and spine is made delightfully flexible, resulting in a more beautiful and youthful YOU!

### Practice schedule

Repeat *The Forehead to Heels Stretch* 3 times at each practice period.

Hold it for 10 seconds during the first week.

Add 5 seconds each week until you are holding it for 30 seconds.

### Special hints

I cannot praise this exercise too highly for beauty as well as health. It is one that you can and should do throughout the day whenever you feel tense or fatigued besides practicing it as part of your regular Yoga period. That minute or so which it takes to perform will repay you many times in terms of freedom from accumulated tension and renewed energy.

Close your eyes when you perform this exercise so that you can feel the delightful relief from tension that it brings.

Always lie down for a few moments after each set of exercises. This is very essential so that you can give these techniques time to replenish your reservoir of vitality. It is also important, as you will experience after you do 3 of these *Forehead to Heel Stretches,* so that you can feel the effects and enjoy their delightful sensation. You will be moulded into a more radiant YOU!

## Exercise 11: THE SPREAD LEG STRETCH

FLEXIBILITY, VITALITY AND ENDURANCE OF
THE LEGS INCREASED. LEGS SLIMMED.

### How to practice this exercise

1. Sit on your mat with your legs extended straight out in front of you, toes and heels together.

2. Without bending your knees spread your legs as far apart as you can. Place one hand, palm down, on the top of each thigh (Fig. 27).

3. Slide your hands forward down your legs until your arms are straight. Then, in the same slow-motion pace, continue sliding your hands down your legs while you bend forward with your upper body as far as you can without strain or discomfort.

4. When you can stretch no further, grasp with your hands whatever part of your extended legs they have reached.

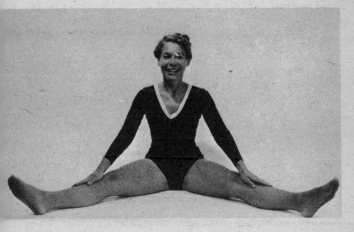

*Figure 27*

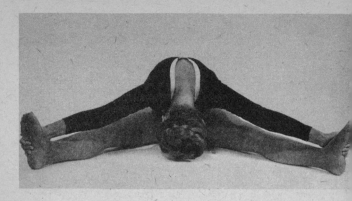

*Figure 28*

5. Have your grip bend your elbows very slowly until you canno comfortably stretch any further. At this point close your eyes and hold the posture motionless for 10 seconds. Fig. 28 shows the advanced stage of this marvelous stretch.

6. To come up out of this posture, first straighten your elbows. Then, releasing your grip, allow your hands to slide back up your legs as your spine slowly straightens up. Your back should "curl" back up rather than straighten up immediately from the waist. Your head should thus be the last part of your trunk to resume an upright position.

7. Rest for a moment in this position and then repeat the exercise for the prescribed number of times.

### Benefits to you

1. The legs are stretched, limbered, firmed up and relieved from the tension that has accumulated in various parts of them.

2. This posture helps trim excessive weight from the thighs.

3. Flabbiness is removed from the thighs and a firm muscle tone appears in its place.

4. The back and spine are made limber and elastic.

5. Circulation is improved in the head and face, natural coloring improves.

6. A general bodily relaxation and invigoration occurs, softening those tired lines.

### Practice schedule

Do *The Spread Leg Stretch* 3 times at each sitting.
Begin by holding it for 10 seconds during the first week.

Add 5 seconds each week until you are holding the posture motionless for 30 seconds.

If you wish to increase the time beyond 30 seconds, you may advance to 60 seconds at the same rate of increase but you need only repeat the exercise twice.

## Special hints

In this posture it is essential that you do not make abrupt movements nor pull or tug in any way that can put a strain upon the muscles and tendons that are being stretched. Enjoy the delightful stretching sensation, but do not attempt to compete with yourself in an effort to attain flexibility faster.

Do not fidget when you are holding this posture nor attempt by adjusting your body, no matter how slightly, to increase your stretch. Simply getting into it and holding it with an enjoyable stretching sensation is enough. Your body will do the rest by itself. In the Western world we attempt to interfere with, to push, and to force nature far too much. Rather, we must realize that our true relationship with nature is at most to help it along by coming to understand how it works and what it is doing. When one understands the way of nature then one realizes that it need only be "helped along" in a very gentle manner by moving harmoniously with it.

Your body is a part of nature. You cannot tell your kidneys what to do or tell your blood how it should absorb oxygen from the air. You cannot command yourself to stop breathing and if you could, you could not command yourself to begin again. You cannot make yourself stop growing or once having stopped make yourself start again. All the functions of your body are a part of nature and, as with nature, they work by themselves. They know what to do if only they are left alone in conditions that are natural and positive for them to work in.

Our job then is to provide nature with the best conditions in which it can function. That is what we are doing in Yoga. We are placing our bodies in positions that are most advantageous to aiding development and proper functioning. Therefore, when you place yourself in one of these stretching positions you should go only as far as enjoyment and relaxation permit. Then, become still and allow your body with its strange and mysterious reservoir of intelligence, to do the rest by itself. And it will—to perfection—if aided in the manner I have intimated.

Breathe quietly and in a relaxed manner while in this posture. Let your neck be limp with your head hanging toward the mat between your knees.

Come out of the posture as slowly and as carefully as you go into it, taking at least 10 seconds to do so.

# CHAPTER TWELVE

# Beauty and Health for the Hips

*About the Hips*

In the realm of beauty there is a mild controversy regarding the subject of women's hips. The current high fashion style has exploited the appearance of women who happen to have slim hips to such an extent that the average woman has come to feel that here is the correct model which they should strive to emulate. The implication of this trend *is* that women who possess slim hips—or even boyish hips, or none at all— are supposed to be considered generally more beautiful and more desirable by men. This is highly debatable. A question often raised is: For whom should women strive to bring out their beauty; for men, for other women, or to live up to transient style established by "authorities" whose business is to sell beauty products?

The answer is that *of these three* the beauty standard involving men would seem to be the most valid one. Here at least there is the purpose of a woman's care and interest in developing her latent beauty and in revealing her appearance to the best possible advantage. She is corresponding to the way of nature, in which the sexes by instinct tend to make themselves attractive for each other.

There are other motives behind why a woman would want to possess the most beautiful possible figure and condition. The motives in general are:

1. Confidence and self-assurance.

2. For reasons of feeling and being healthy.

(There is rarely a natural and real beauty without the corresponding natural and real health.)

3. To be attractive to men.

(Strong protestation to the contrary should be subject to equally strong self-examination from a psychological point of view. We hear much in our sophisticated times how women dress, for example, for other women. One cannot exactly call this a normal, wholesome, balanced state of mind, nor a courageous one.)

4. Finally, for self respect.

(It is no tribute to normal, healthy human pride for a woman to allow herself to fall so badly out of shape that she loses the beauty that is hers and becomes drab, oppressive to the sight, grotesque or worse. There is a natural joy in looking one's best to the world and it need not be vanity.)

Our theme has been that the shape that is yours when you are at the peak of normal health is the only ideal figure or standard toward which you should ever strive. If nature has given you a basically shapely, curvaceous form with hips that might even be termed ample, then consider yourself as fortunate as women who possess any other type of figure. Your goal is to bring out *your* figure. If you attain the degree of health and physical fitness that is potentially yours and which can be easily attained through Yoga, then you yourself will be a living standard of beauty.

## Exercise 12: THE HALF LOCUST

HIPS SLENDERIZED AND MADE FIRM.

### How to practice this exercise

1. Lie on your abdomen on your mat with your hands at your sides, your face resting on one cheek and your toes together. Become completely limp in this position (Fig. 29).

2. Bring your heels together so that both toes and heels are now together with the toes extended outward away from your body. Clench your hands into fists and place your fists thumbs down closely against your sides. Turn your head and rest your chin against the mat somewhat more toward your lower lip than towards the point of your chin (Fig. 30).

3. Slowly raise your left leg as high into the air as you can. Aid the lifting of your leg by pushing downward with your fists against the mat. Do not bend your upraised leg at the knee (Fig. 31).

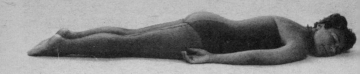

*Figure 29*

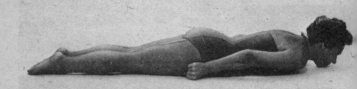

*Figure 30*

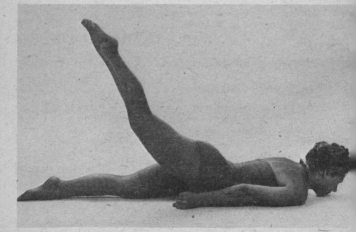

*Figure 31*

4. Hold this position for 10 seconds. Breathe normally and count the seconds to yourself.

5. Slowly lower your leg, taking at least 10 seconds to do so.

6. When both legs are once again on the floor, rest as limply as you can for a few moments.

7. Repeat the same movement raising the alternate leg (Fig. 32).

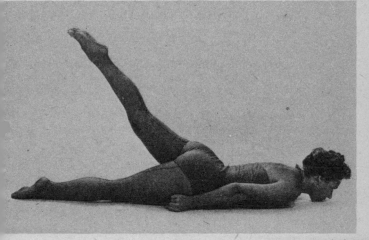

*Figure 32*

### Benefits to you

1. *The Half Locust* firms and strengthens the hips, buttocks, and thighs.

2. It aids in reducing weight in these areas.

3. It stimulates circulation through vital visceral organs such as the liver, intestines, kidneys and reproductive glands and organs.

4. It strengthens the abdomen and the muscles of the lower back.

5. It is a splendid workout for the seldom used muscles of the pelvic region, toning them for a svelte figure.

### Practice schedule

Do *The Half Locust* posture 3 times on each leg, alternating your legs. For example, first raise your left leg, then your right, then left, etc.

For the first week hold your upraised leg motionless for 10 seconds.

Add 5 seconds to your holding time each week until you are holding it for 30 seconds.

### Special hints

If you especially enjoy this technique, you may continue to increase the holding time by 5 seconds each week. This is a mild technique and cannot be overdone providing you adhere to the specified rate of increasing your holding time.

*The Half Locust* has a two-fold function. First, it is a therapeutic exercise in itself. Second, it is a preparatory exercise for *The Full Locust*. Therefore, when you begin to become efficient in *The Full Locust*, in which you will be instructed shortly and which is a more difficult exercise, it is more important for you to practice *The Full Locust* than *The Half Locust*.

It is essential to keep your upraised leg straight in this posture. You will only be cheating yourself out of its many benefits if you bend your leg.

Remember to come down out of the posture very slowly, taking at least 10 seconds to do so. It is a very graceful and lovely technique and you should be aware of the gracefulness as you perform it. It can condition you for grace in all body movements.

## Exercise 13: THE ANKLE TO FOREHEAD STRETCH

A SCIENTIFIC STRETCHING OF THE HIP AREA.

### How to practice this technique

1. Sit down on your mat with your legs extended straight out in front of you, toes and heels together. Bend your right leg at the knee and bring your right foot toward you so that you can grasp it with your hands.

2. Take your right hand and place it underneath your ankle approximately over the region of your outer ankle bone.

3. Grasp your right foot with your left hand holding it with a firm grip around the arch (Fig. 33).

4. Using the strength of your arms and bending your head forward as far as balance will permit, lift your right leg up drawing your ankle toward your forehead.

5. When you have either reached your forehead with the inside of your ankle or have brought your ankle as close to your forehead as you comfortably can, hold this stretching position for 5 seconds (Fig. 34 and Fig. 35).

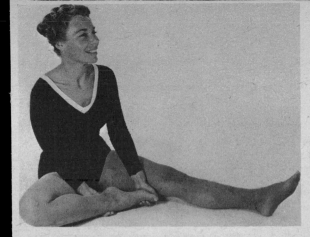

*Figure 33*

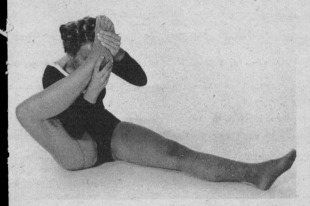

*Figure 34*

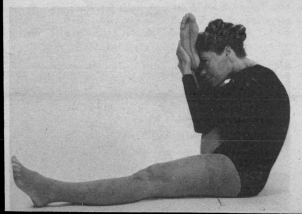

*Figure 35*

6. Very slowly, *as in all Yoga exercises,* lower your leg back to the ground.

7. Stretch your right leg out in front of you and then perform the same movement with the other leg.

### Benefits to you

1. The muscles and connective tissue of the hips are stretched, toned, and firmed.

2. The *Ankle to Forehead Stretch* is wonderfully therapeutic for the hip joints. It is a form of self applied chiropractic treatment and is of special benefit for the great sciatic nerve.

3. *The Ankle to Forehead Stretch* gives greater flexibility to the legs, and beautifies them.

4. Strength in the arms is developed.

### Practice schedule

Perform this exercise 3 times on each leg, alternating legs from left to right to left, etc.

Begin by holding the posture for 5 seconds during the first week. Add 3 seconds each week until you are holding it for 20 seconds.

### Special hints

Many people will not be able to reach their ankle with their forehead in the beginning, indicating an unnatural tightness and stiffness in the hips, and in the muscular area where the thighs and buttocks meet. Simply bring your foot as far as you can toward your forehead and hold your stretch at its farthest point. As with all Yoga exercises your body will "give" in time and you will regain your normal flexibility and all the healthful results that come with it.

The main thing is to reach your ankle to your forehead. If at first you must bend your head considerably forward in order to enable this meeting to take place, do so. Later you will be able to perform the posture with your back held correctly in a more erect position.

Once you do attain contact between ankle and forehead, hold it firmly.

# CHAPTER THIRTEEN

# Beauty and Health
# for the Buttocks

*About the Buttocks*

The main danger to the esthetic appearance of the buttocks is excessive weight. Also, as time goes by, those muscles grow flabby and tend to sag. The function of exercise regarding this area is to keep the muscles firm and as shapely as common sense and the limitations of one's age and natural figure permits.

Besides the Yoga techniques which work both directly and indirectly on this area and restore it to its healthiest condition, there are other steps which I would also recommend. Due to the difficulty of bringing this area back up to a normal, healthful and esthetic condition once it has begun to deteriorate, the best advice is to keep off it as much as you are able. Sitting around too much or an inactive way of life in general will contribute to its becoming excessively heavy, flabby and out of shape. If, however, you happen to have a sedentary occupation, I recommend that you apply yourself sincerely to the Yoga exercises that relate directly to the buttocks as well as to areas adjacent to the buttocks such as the waist and the thighs. You should also walk whenever possible instead of ride. We are very spoiled these days. It is tragic to note that the average person gets into a car to drive three or four blocks. Actually a three- or four-block walk is barely a warm up for the normal human body.

## How to Walk with Beauty Benefits

A ten-block walk is a short walk. To begin to do some good you should walk whenever possible. Do not walk as if it were a chore with the idea that you are lugging your body somewhere as you would a heavy suitcase. Walk vigorously with your chest up and out, breathing rhythmically. When I walk I breathe in for eight steps and out for eight steps, establishing a rhythm much as swimmers use which enables them to swim for very long distances and not be tired. You can, as well, simply breathe deeply and fully as you walk. Walk briskly with long healthy strides. Realize that walking is one of the finest forms of exercise when correctly executed. It has a direct effect on helping to firm and trim the buttocks.

## Other Exercises for Beauty Benefits

*Swimming* is another exercise I recommend which, besides its universally known therapeutic effect upon the total body, also has a direct effect upon reducing flabbiness in the buttocks. *Bicycle riding* is also a superlative exercise for that area. Now remember that a bicycle ride once around the block is not going to do very much. While it may sound extreme to think of riding a bicycle for one or two miles, you will find that a one- or two-mile bicycle ride is little more than a matter of a few minutes and is wonderfully exhilarating.

Remember also that housework can have two aspects. It can either be an unpleasant drudgery or it can be a wonderful form of exercise, which, like walking, swimming and bicycle riding can augment your Yoga exercise program. *The important thing is to do your housework as pleasurable exercise.* When you bend down, bend as if you are bending toward your toes. If you carry something, carry it with your chest out and use those muscles. Don't make it a chore. You will find that it can have tremendous effects upon helping to slim down various portions of your body and it will do much to transform drudgery into a kind of healthful game.

The buttocks are a difficult part of the body to keep under control weightwise. Weight tends to accumulate in certain parts of the body first in different people. Some women collect weight in their thighs before any other part. In some it accumulates in the abdomen or around the waist. With others it is around the buttocks. The exercise you are going to learn next is superlative for keeping the buttocks firm and for controlling weight in that area. You must, of course, realize that you cannot practice Yoga haphazardly and expect to attain results. You must practice these exercises regularly and correctly every day and according to the practice schedule given with each exercise.

### Exercise 14: THE LOCUST POSTURE

TIGHTENS, FIRMS AND REDUCES WEIGHT IN THE
BUTTOCKS.

#### *How to practice this exercise*

1. Lie on your abdomen on your mat.
2. Extend your toes straight out and bring your heels and toes
together. Clench your hands into fists and place your fists thumbs down
closely against your sides. Turn your head so that your chin rests upon
the mat, but closer to your lower lip than to the point of your chin. This
is the starting position (Fig. 36).

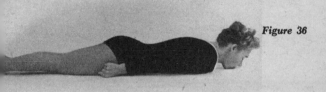

Figure 36

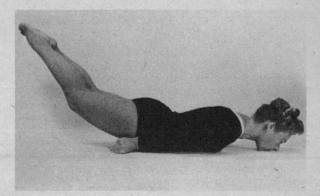

igure 37

3. Inhale approximately a half-lungful of air. Retain this air in your lungs throughout the entire exercise.

4. As soon as you have inhaled as instructed, tighten your entire body and, helping yourself by pushing downward with your arms, raise both legs up into the air as high as you can.

5. Hold your legs up in the air in this position for 5 seconds (Fig. 37).

6. As slowly and as controlled as you can, lower your legs back down onto the floor.

7. Exhale your breath in a controlled manner not allowing it to gush out forcefully.

8. Turn your face onto your cheek and go completely limp from head to toes. Rest this way for several moments.

9. Repeat the exercise in exactly the same manner.

### Benefits to you

1. *The Locust* strengthens the muscles of the buttocks, lower back, abdomen and thighs.

2. It trims and firms the hips and buttocks.

3. It helps reduce weight in the buttocks, hips and thighs.

4. It improves blood circulation especially in the vital organs of the abdominal cavity for the glow of health.

5. *The Locust* is a beneficial exercise for the sexual glands and organs.

### Practice schedule

Do *The Locust* 3 times at each practice period.

Hold your highest position for 3 seconds during the first week.

Add only 1 second each week to your holding time until you are able to hold *The Locust* for 10 seconds.

### Special hints

Besides the remarkable effects that *The Locust* has upon the internal organs and upon firming and reshaping the body from the waist to the thighs, it is also a strengthening posture. It increases the strength in your legs, abdomen, and lower back, giving that lean, supple look.

As with all the Yoga techniques, do not be deceived by the simplicity of their execution. *The Locust,* for example, is extremely powerful in its effects. Of all the Yoga exercises you will be taught, *The Locust* is the one requiring the greatest amount of physical effort on your part. It is indeed the only Yoga technique that borders upon being somewhat strenuous. You will perhaps find it difficult to perform in the beginning, but have patience and persevere because its effects upon you are so wonderful.

Remember to keep your thumbs against the floor and your fists closely against your sides. Always lower your legs as slowly as you can. You may, in this particular instance, cheat a little; that is, if you feel that you can get up a little higher in the beginning weeks and hold *The Locust* a little steadier, you may bend your legs *slightly* at the knees. The sooner you can perform *The Locust* with your knees straight, however, the greater will be its effects upon you.

Remember to place your chin a bit closer to your lower lip rather than on the point of it. Do not collapse out of this posture, either in coming down with your legs or with the expulsion of your breath, no matter how much you might be tempted.

When you go up into *The Locust,* try to throw your body weight onto your chin and arms.

The words discipline and self-control have become nearly bad words for too many people. This is unfortunate because, as you will experience in Yoga, self-control is one of the most exciting challenges that any person can accept. Rather than being "work" the discipline of Yoga is more of a delightful game which one plays with oneself. The mere sitting down and performing of these Yoga techniques is in itself a *triumph of control over your body*. Its effect upon your bearing, your health, your appearance, and upon all the other activities of your life will be noticeable even from the beginning as you develop your hidden beauty!

# CHAPTER FOURTEEN

# Beauty and Health
# for the Abdomen

## About the Abdomen

Softness, sagging, protrusion and overweight are the most common problems relating to the abdomen. Difficulties in this area regarding overweight and deteriorated muscle tone are not hard to solve. The abdomen responds quickly to correct physical exercise.

Of course these problems are not to be treated lightly. Deterioration of the abdomen reflects grave danger to the health. When an abdomen is overweight or protruding because the abdominal wall has lost its muscle tone, the internal organs that are held in place by the abdominal muscles become misplaced. They sag with the wall. This is a very serious condition because an organ that is sagging out of its normal place in the abdominal cavity cannot function in a proper manner. In addition to endangering your health, a sagging, protruding or overweight abdomen is extremely unsightly and, in fact, after a certain point, is a decidedly revolting sight to behold.

A slight feminine curvature, however, is in a great percentage of cases normal as well as esthetic. The current flat abdomen mania is not wholesome or right when applied to a woman whose basic body type and bone structure does not by nature require it. Some women are naturally curvaceous with full hips, full bosoms and full calves. Such women will tend to have a slight curvature of the abdomen. In this case it would be decidedly unnatural and negative for them to attempt to force their abdomen to be as flat as that of let us say an essentially slender, thin-boned woman.

You should strive only to attain the best physical condition possible for your basic body structure. All this requires of the abdomen is that it be firm and strong. If there is a moderate natural rotundity of the abdomen in individual cases, and, if a woman is in her best physical condition, she will feel her best, appear at her loveliest and her vital abdominal glands and organs will be held high and in their proper healthful place.

### Exercise 15: THE PLOUGH

STRENGTHENS, TIGHTENS, AND ELIMINATES EXCESSIVE WEIGHT IN THE ABDOMINAL AREA.

*How to practice this exercise*

1. Lie on your mat on your back. Allow your body to become completely limp from toes to head (Fig. 38).

2. Bring your heels and toes together. Turn your hands so that your palms rest on the floor close to your sides (Fig. 39).

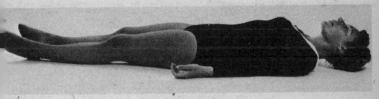

*Figure 38*

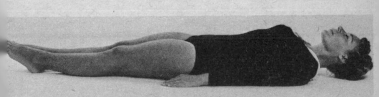

*Figure 39*

3. Tighten your abdomen and legs and, as slowly as you can, raise your legs straight up in the air until they are at a ninety degree angle to the rest of your body. Do not bend your knees. Help yourself raise your legs in this manner by pressing downward against the floor with your hands. You should attempt to take at least 10 seconds to raise your legs to the vertical position (Fig. 40).

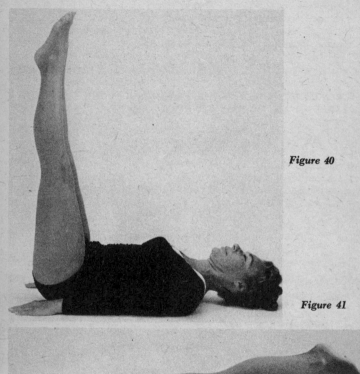

*Figure 40*

*Figure 41*

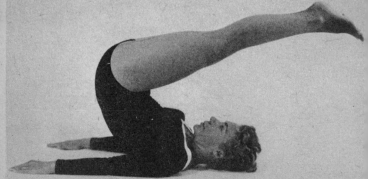

4. Helping yourself once again by pushing against the floor with your hands, raise your buttocks and lower back off the floor so that your legs come over your body toward your head (Fig. 41).

5. Continue going backward toward your head with your legs but bend your body at the waist so that your feet move downward toward the floor behind your head.

NOTE: If you cannot stretch back far enough for your toes to touch the floor behind your head, simply go as far as you comfortably can and hold your farthest position for the prescribed number of seconds. As time goes by—and it does not take long in this exercise—the stiff muscles and tendons of your back and spine will "give" as they regain their normal flexibility. The sheer weight of your legs will cause this to happen, stretching your back and spine and other stiff areas in a natural, wholesome and wonderfully delightful manner. Never attempt to force this or any other posture nor to bob up and down in an attempt to reach the floor with your toes. The stretch will take place naturally by itself.

6. When your toes have reached the floor behind your head, hold that position for 5 seconds (Fig. 42).

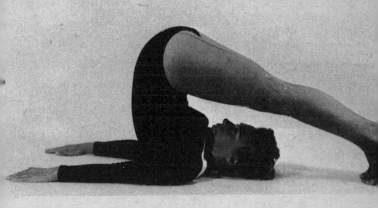

*Figure 42*

7. Now slide your hands slowly from their original position up toward your head and carefully clasp them against the *top* of your head (Fig. 43).

8. Hold this position for 5 seconds (Fig. 44).

9. Slide your hands slowly back down to their original position, palms down against the floor and brace yourself with them.

10. Slowly bend your legs at the knees, bringing your knees to within an inch or two from your face (Fig. 45).

11. Keeping the back of your head against the floor at all times, allow your body to come slowly forward until your lower back rests once again comfortably on the floor (Figs. 46 and 47).

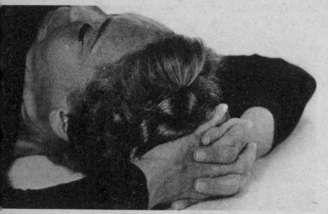

Figure 43

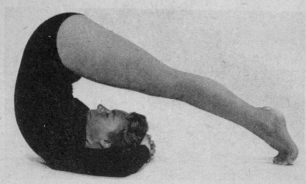

Figure 44

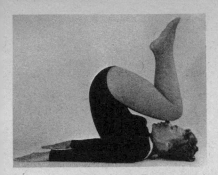

Figure 45

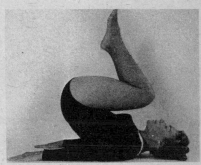

Figure 46

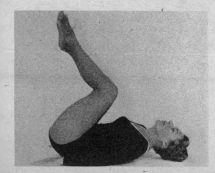

Figure 47

NOTE: It is essential to keep your head against the floor at all times while coming out of this posture. If you do not you will lose control and roll quickly out of it, thus breaking the posture and detracting from a great many of its results. By keeping your head against the floor and controlling the forward movement of your body by applying pressure against the floor with your hands, you will in a very few days gain complete control of your coming out of *The Plough* and you will come out of it in a slow-motion forward roll which is both healthful and graceful.

12. When your lower back and buttocks rest upon the floor, straighten your legs extending them straight up into the air so that they are once again at a ninety degree angle to your body.

13. As slowly as you can, taking at least 10 seconds to do so, lower your legs back down to the floor. Do not bend your knees (Fig. 48). If you are able, when your legs are a few inches from the floor, stop lowering them and attempt to hold them still for as long as you can. This greatly drives home the effects of this exercise upon your abdomen.

14. Let your body become completely limp and rest this way for at least 30 seconds after coming out of *The Plough*.

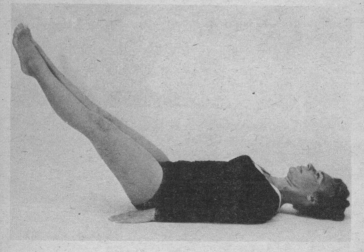

*Figure 48*

### Benefits to you

1. *The Plough* strengthens the muscles of the abdomen.
2. It reduces weight in the abdomen.
3. It massages, stimulates and manipulates vital internal organs in the abdominal region such as the kidneys, liver, spleen, and intestines.
4. It helps to firm and trim the thighs and hips.
5. It helps reduce general body weight because of its effect upon the thyroid gland.
6. *The Plough* relieves deep tension that has become accumulated and hidden in the back, neck and in the great tendons of the legs and toes.
7. You will feel a surge of new vitality come through your entire body after performing this posture because of the tension that has been removed throughout your back, spine, neck and legs. Tension drains vitality. Thus when tension is removed your natural vital force can flow through you undiminished.
8. *The Plough* imparts great elasticity and limberness to the spinal column.
9. It strengthens the neck.
10. Due to the increased circulation throughout the head that is produced by this exercise, the complexion tends to be very much improved. In India *The Plough* is prescribed medically for the treatment of many skin disorders of the face.
11. Circulation is stimulated and improved throughout the brain itself, refreshing the brain and giving the student a new-found alertness of the mind and senses.
12. Scores upon scores of students throughout the years have told me about the ability of *The Plough* to relieve headaches.

### Practice schedule

Do *The Plough* as instructed 3 times at each workout. This is a very important Yoga exercise and I cannot overstate its general healthful effect upon the body.

Hold each position as instructed for 5 seconds during the first week.

Add 5 seconds to each one every week until you are holding each position for 20 seconds.

At this point you may, if you wish, eliminate the first position and go directly into the second position where your hands are clasped on top of your head. Upon doing so you should increase the holding time of that second position alone by 5 seconds each week until you are holding it for 45 seconds.

### Special hints

Rest for at least 30 seconds limply after each time that you do *The Plough*. Rest for at least one full minute after you have performed it for the third time.

If you feel any shortness of breath in the beginning do not be perplexed. This is a normal phenomenon in the first few days or weeks of performing the posture. In a very short time your breath will adjust itself and you will be breathing slowly and normally in it.

Do not bend your knees at any time while you are performing *The Plough* except in the first stage of coming out of it as instructed. Do not make any abrupt or jerky movements of your body while in the posture. Practice "being still" which in itself is a valuable physical and mental discipline.

*The Plough* has tremendous ability to streamline the body. It is so relaxing that it gives to the student a feeling, tone and aura of great physical and mental serenity.

The spine has been compressed by unnatural use for many years. It has a nearly incredible ability to stretch and it needs to be stretched if you want to experience and possess that natural health and vibrance which is your birthright. Even if you cannot get into the final position of *The Plough* right away, practice holding it at the farthest point that you can comfortably reach and you will experience for yourself how your vertebrae will relax and stretch.

As to the raising of your lower back and buttocks from the floor when first going up and over into *The Plough*, you must accomplish this by whatever means necessary. You can rock for a while and give yourself a great push if you need to do so in order to raise your posterior from the floor.

Remember your hands are clasped on "top" of your head and not "under" your head at the base of your skull. Observe the photograph carefully.

# CHAPTER FIFTEEN

# Beauty and Health for the Waist

*About the Waist*

Overweight and thickness are the main problems of the waist. The solution to these problems and to the problems of most body parts and areas is "use." The proper use of the waist is scientific twisting and bending. The Yoga techniques that directly affect the waist are made all the more effective when used in conjunction with Yoga exercises that slim the abdomen and normalize body weight.

A big woman, no matter what her present condition or proportions, can increase her beauty and appeal one hundred fold right away by reducing her waist. Women who may be generally just a bit too curvaceous and who have difficulty in reducing other parts of their body quickly (such as the thighs and hips) can become years younger and look more attractive while they continue to work on the rest of their body simply by reducing excess weight in their waist.

### Exercise 16: THE TWIST

HELPS SLIM THE WAIST.

*How to practice this exercise*

1. Sit on your mat with both legs extended straight out in front of you, heels and toes together. Your back is erect.

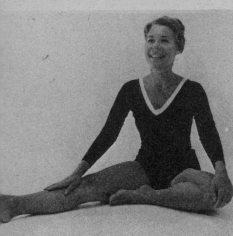

Figure 49

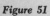

Figure 51

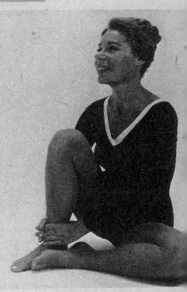

Figure 50

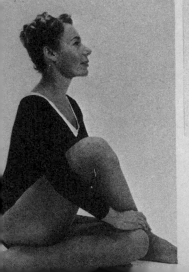

2. Bend your left leg at the knee and bring it toward your body so that you can grasp it with your hands.

3. Place the sole of your left foot against (not under) the inside of your right thigh with your left heel as close to your groin as possible. Your left knee is against or near the floor (Fig. 49).

4. Bend your right leg at the knee but this time keep your right knee up in the air. Bring your right foot toward you so that you can grasp it with both hands.

5. Take your right foot in your hands and place it sole down upon the floor so that the soles of both feet are next to each other (Fig. 50).

6. Grasp your right ankle with your hands and slowly lift your right foot up and carry it over your left knee. Having done this, place the sole of your right foot on the floor on the left side of your left knee (Fig. 51).

7. Take your right hand and place it palm down on the floor by your right side slightly behind you. This is to balance your body during the next movements.

8. Bend your left arm at the elbow and hook the elbow over your right knee (Fig. 52).

9. Straighten your left arm out until you grasp your left knee with your left hand. If you have difficulty grasping your knee, you may take hold of any part of your left leg that you can reach (Fig. 53).

10. Now lift your right arm into the air in front of you, elbow straight. Focus your eyes on your fingertips.

11. Slowly move your right arm around to your right with your eyes still focused upon your fingertips so that your head follows your arm in its smooth turn to the right (Fig. 54).

12. When you can no longer move your arm to the right, bend it at the elbow and bring it around behind you so that your right hand clasps the left side of your waist. Your head is now twisted around to your right as far as it can go. Your eyes are looking to the right as far as they can (Fig. 55).

13. Hold this twisting position for 10 seconds counting the time slowly to yourself. (See Fig. 56 for correct hand position behind back.)

14. To come out of *The Twist* first drop your right arm slowly until it is resting once again palm down on the floor behind you. Then, slowly turn your head back to a forward position. When this part of the stretch is relieved, carefully and gently release your left hand from your left knee. Bring your right hand forward and grasp your right ankle with both hands. Lift your right foot over your left knee once again until it is back in position of Fig. 50. Straighten your right leg out. Then straighten your left leg out until you are sitting with both legs before you ready to repeat the exercise.

15. Repeat *The Twist*, only each time do so on a different side.

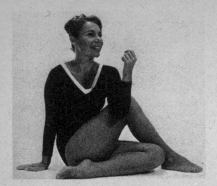

*Figure 52*

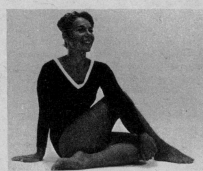

*Figure 53*

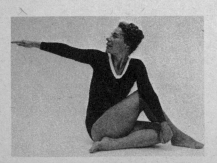

*Figure 54*

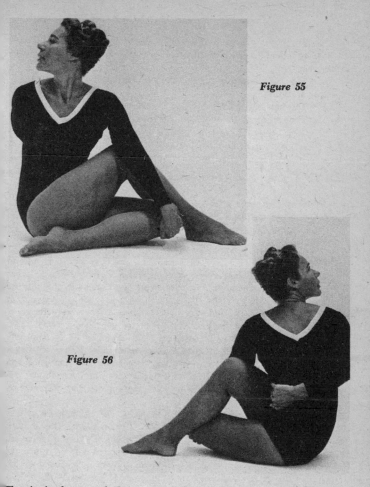

Figure 55

Figure 56

That is, in the second *Twist* you will bend your right leg and place the sole of your right foot against the inside of your left thigh, etc.

### Benefits to you

1. *The Twist* is a great aid in reducing weight in the waist and in restoring its sleek trim look.

2. Every vertebra of the spinal column is stretched individually by this exercise in a spiral or twisting direction. It has a marvelously relaxing effect on the nervous system.

101

3. *The Twist* relieves deep tension in the back and spine.

4. It removes tension in the neck and adjusts the vertebrae in the neck area.

5. *The Twist* improves the posture and is a mild corrective for many postural disorders.

6. The hip joint is limbered and stretched.

7. The muscles of the shoulders are toned.

### Practice schedule

Do *The Twist* 3 times on each side. Alternate the sides from right to left to right to left to right to left.

Begin by holding *The Twist* motionless in your farthest position for 10 seconds on each side.

Add 5 seconds each week until you are holding it for 30 seconds.

### Special hints

*The Twist* is a slightly complicated Yoga exercise but it is fun and the sensation you will experience once your body begins to become limber in it is absolutely delightful. The body happens to adapt to this posture very quickly and you will be thrilled at how soon you will slip into it effortlessly. It is a gentle and very scientific stretch for every vertebra of your spinal column and for every other part of your body related to it.

*The Twist,* as is the case with all Yoga exercises, is a completely natural movement and natural position for your body. Your body loves these postures and, in fact, craves doing them. You will find once you begin to limber up in several of these exercises that your body will demand that you sit down and relieve the tension that has accumulated in it by performing them.

*The Twist* is a most ingenious movement. For example, as it was instructed here, the left arm locks the right leg in place. This in turn locks the lower portion of the spine so that it is held in a forward position. Against this stationary base you twist the entire spinal column in a corkscrew direction. Every vertebra of your spine is given a controlled stretch much like the pressure on each individual link if you were to hold a chain in a vertical position and twist it in opposite directions at each end.

Make sure you keep your head up as erectly as you can when performing *The Twist*.

Your breath may be a bit short in the beginning but in a very few days it will adjust itself and you will be breathing normally throughout the posture.

A very important point concerns the eyes. Throughout the actual holding of *The Twist* it is the eyes that make certain that the posture is held tightly and that you do not slip out of it inadvertently. In whatever direction your head is turning you must make sure that your eyes are looking to that corner of their sockets. Your eyes are, in a way, directing the entire twist as they follow your hand. If your head is twisted, for example, to the right, your eyes should be in the extreme right side of their sockets. As soon as you look forward with them while holding *The Twist* you are in danger of loosening the entire stretch and thus losing much of its benefits.

The foot that rests upon its sole during *The Twist* (such as the right foot in Fig. 51), is a kind of adjusting lever for the posture. The placement of this foot adjusts and alters the difficulty of the stretch. The further away from your body the foot is, the easier it is to get into *The Twist*. Thus if a person has a large stomach or is overweight in certain other areas that obstruct this particular exercise, he may feel free at first to move the foot forward away from the body so that he can twist around more easily. On the other hand as you become proficient in *The Twist*— and you will, sooner than you can imagine—you may wish to increase the intensity of the stretch. To do this simply pull the foot on the outside of your base leg closer to your body.

People who have unusual difficulty in getting into *The Twist* because of such reasons as age, stiffness, or overweight may use the leg position shown in Fig. 57 where the legs are simply crossed lightly one over the other on the floor. Other than this simple crossing of the legs the rest of the posture is done in exactly the same manner as instructed.

Another variation, or a simpler way of performing *The Twist*, is to

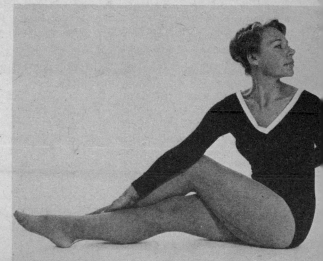

*Figure 57*

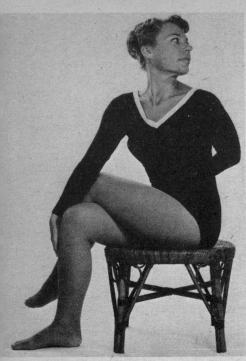

*Figure 58*

do so with your legs crossed while sitting in a chair as in Fig. 58. This variation is especially suitable for elderly persons or for people who have some sort of disability which would prevent them from using their legs in the regular way. Do not use these two variations unless it is really necessary.

### Exercise 17: THE SIDE BENDS

TIGHTENS AND SLIMS THE WAIST.

*How to practice this exercise*

1. Stand erectly with your hands at your sides and your feet at approximately shoulder width (Fig. 59).

2. Raise your arms slowly out from your sides until they are extended sideways, elbows straight, at shoulder level (Fig. 60).

3. Bend slowly to your right side taking at least 10 seconds to reach your farthest position.

4. When you have stretched to the point where you can go no farther comfortably, hold that position motionless for 10 seconds (Fig. 61).

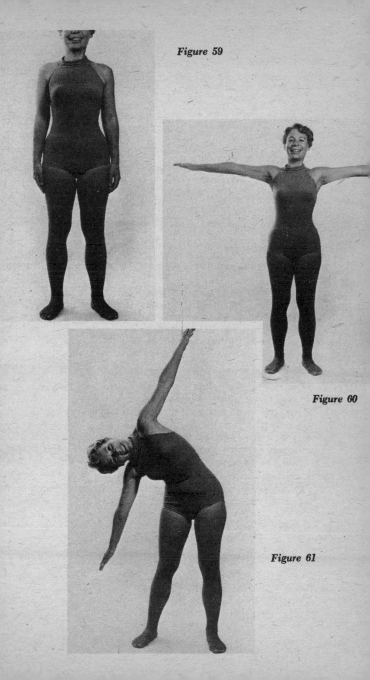

Figure 59

Figure 60

Figure 61

5. Employing the same slow motion that you used going into your stretch, straighten up out of it until you are once more standing erectly with your arms extended outward from your sides.

6. Lower your arms slowly to your sides.

7. Perform the exact same movement bending toward the *left* side.

### Benefits to you

1. *The Side Bends* reduce weight in the waist.

2. Seldom used muscles of the thighs are toned, making them firm and taut.

3. The relatively weak muscles of the sides are strengthened and tension is removed by stretching.

4. The spine is given a healthful sideways stretch.

### Practice schedule

Do *The Side Bends* 3 times on each side alternating the sides from right to left.

Begin by holding your farthest position for 10 seconds.

Add 5 seconds each week until you are holding the stretch motionless for 30 seconds. At this point if your waist is not a major problem to you and time compels you to abbreviate your workout, you may perform the stretching posture only twice on each side.

### Special hints

When you go down into the stretch toward your side, allow your head to hang down with your neck limp.

Keep your knees straight at all times throughout the exercise. You will feel a stretch in various portions of your legs as you become more limber in it. You will detract from the results if you bend your knees.

Remember to keep your sideward bend strictly toward the side and *do not lean forward toward the front*. This is a frequent error that occurs during practice.

*The Side Bends* are splendid to do whenever the pressures of the day mount up. It is a technique that you can feel free to perform at any spare time whenever you have a moment of privacy.

## Exercise 18: VARIATION OF THE ALTERNATE LEG PULL

AN ADVANCED POSTURE FOR KEEPING WEIGHT
OFF THE WAIST AND THIGHS.

### How to practice this exercise

1. Sit on your mat in the basic starting position, legs extended straight out in front of you, toes and heels together, your back erect and your chest held high (Fig. 62).

2. Bend your left leg at the knee and with your knee toward or upon the floor bring your left foot toward you so that you can grasp it with both hands.

3. Take your left foot with your hands and place your left sole against the inside of your right thigh with your heel as close to your groin as you can bring it without any strain (Fig. 63).

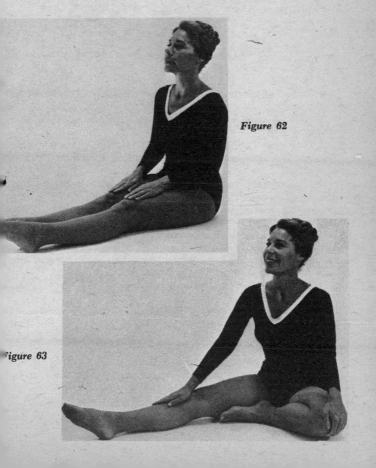

Figure 62

Figure 63

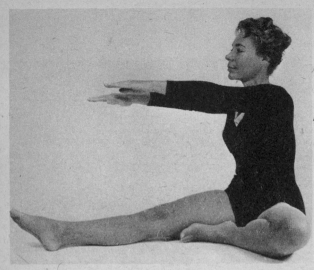

*Figure 64*

4. Slowly raise both arms straight out in front of you until they are extended palms down at eye level.

5. Keeping your elbows straight, cross your left arm over your right arm (Fig. 64).

6. Now bend forward slowly (Fig. 65) with your intention being to grasp the inside of your extended leg wherever you can reach it with your right hand.

7. Twisting your body very slowly and carefully so that the right side of your head and face will be facing your extended right leg, attempt to grasp with your left hand (your left arm will be alongside the left side of your head and face) the outside of your right leg. Stretch only as far as you can and if you cannot reach your leg with your left hand, simply perform the stretch with that hand reaching toward your extended leg as far as is comfortable. Check the proper position of your hands and arms and the proper twist of your body with Fig. 66.

8. Hold your farthest position for 10 seconds. For the complete posture see Fig. 67.

9. Come out of this posture very slowly by (1) allowing yourself to become limp all over, (2) twisting your body back into a normal forward stretching position and (3) sliding your hands back up your extended leg until you are sitting upright once again.

10. Straighten your left leg until both legs are out in front of you. Repeat the posture on the other side by first bending your right leg and placing the sole of your right foot against the inside of your left thigh, etc.

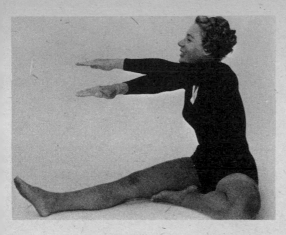

Figure 65

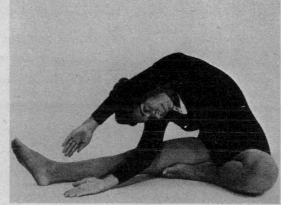

Figure 66

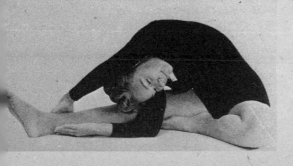

Figure 67

### Benefits to you

1. This posture is a powerful trimmer of excess weight from the waist.

2. It is a splendid stretch for the legs, restoring youthful limberness to them.

3. It helps reduce hips and thighs.

4. It makes the back flexible and removes tension from the back, sides and legs.

5. Wonderful limberness of the spinal column is developed.

### Practice schedule

Do the *Variation of the Alternate Leg Pull* 2 times on each side, alternating the sides.

Hold your farthest position motionless for 5 seconds during the first week.

Add 5 seconds each week to your holding time until you are holding it for 20 seconds.

### Special hints

This is an advanced and difficult posture. I have included it because of its specific effect upon the waist. Bear in mind that complete flexibility does not come as quickly as it does in most other postures.

Do not make the mistake, however, of changing the wonderful challenge that Yoga holds for you into a kind of work or grimly dutiful operation as regards this particular posture. You should rather play with it, feel your way into it, make a game out of it. Go only as far as you can and enjoy the splendid stretch it gives you.

When your body has adapted to the posture and you begin to attain flexibility in it, you will experience a wonderful sense of accomplishment. In speaking of those very few postures which take a bit longer to accomplish than others, it is important to know that once you do attain flexibility in them, with the expenditure of a mere few minutes each day, you keep that flexibility always. This means that for the rest of your life, by practicing a number of seconds on each one every day, you will be able to retain youthful flexibility of body. This flexibility is your best insurance against becoming a victim of the symptoms of old age.

# CHAPTER SIXTEEN

# Beauty and Health
# for the Back

## *About the Back*

The back constitutes a large area of your body and it is subject to many ills. We are always hearing of back pains, disc trouble, strain, pulled muscles and general aching in that area. Despite the size and bulk of the back muscles, it would appear to be a very delicate region susceptible to many negative conditions.

The reason for this is that the back, like many other body parts, has been misused and allowed to deteriorate through lack of use. Many kinds of work necessitate unnatural movements and are bad for the back. Included are the majority of manual jobs which result in so many strains, sprains and other ailments. Sedentary work is just as bad if not worse as it contracts the spine, making it stiff and inelastic with resulting harmful effects upon the nervous system. It is necessary to do something active and efficient to offset the negative factors in our work and in our daily life that cause back trouble.

## *Your Back Accumulates Tension*

The back is a vast area of accumulated tension. To the overwhelming majority of people the back is full of stiff, tight and tense places by the time they are scarcely out of their teens. This very stiffness and tight-

111

ness is the reason why pulled muscles and slipped discs occur so easily and so frequently.

It is the old story of the oak tree and the bamboo. When excessive strain is put upon an oak tree by, let us say, a strong wind, it will at a certain point break regardless of its bulk or strength. Under the same strain or more the bamboo tree cannot be destroyed or injured because it is flexible and simply gives and bends pliably before the wind. The back that is tight and stiff through lack of proper use or through lack of scientific conditioning is like the oak tree, the slightest unexpected strain and injury results. On the other hand, the back which is limber and elastic through the practice of Yoga can bend pliably in the face of many strains or physical requirements no matter how sudden or unusual they might be.

Besides the health benefits of a limber back, when your back is flexible and tension free you will feel youthful, relaxed, and full of new-found vitality and verve. The more limber and properly conditioned a woman's back becomes, the more sleek, trim and lovely her figure will be.

## Exercise 19: THE COMPLETE LEG AND BACK STRETCH

ADJUSTS THE VERTEBRAE. TONES THE NERVOUS
SYSTEM. RELIEVES TENSION FROM THE BACK.
RESTORES YOUTHFUL LIMBERNESS.

### *How to practice this exercise*

1. Sit on your mat with your legs extended straight out in front of you, your toes and heels together, knees straight and with your back erect and chest held high (Fig. 68).

2. Raise your arms until they are straight up in front of you, elbows straight, palms down and hands at eye level.

3. Lean slightly backwards at the waist (Fig. 69) and then bend slowly forward aiming your hands for the farthest part of your extended legs that you can reach without strain.

4. It should take you at least 10 seconds to reach your farthest point. Grasp whatever part of your legs you are able to reach. It may be your toes, feet, ankles, calves, knees or thighs depending upon how stiff you are (Fig. 70).

5. Having a firm grip on your legs, bend your arms very gently and slowly at the elbows and pull yourself down until you have reached your limit (Fig. 71).

Fig. 72 represents the ultimate stretch in this posture. The head rests on the knees, the fingers grasp the toes and the elbows touch the floor.

6. Now close your eyes, let your neck become limp, aim your head toward your knees, breathe normally and hold the position motionless for 10 seconds.

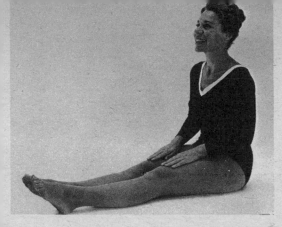

Figure 68

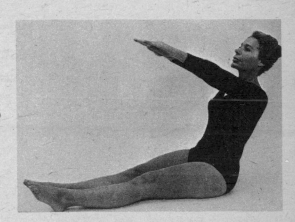

Figure 69

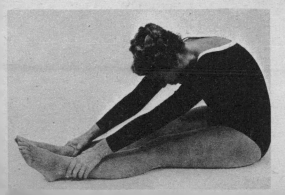

Figure 70

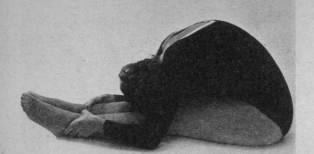

*Figure 71*

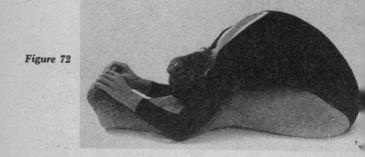

*Figure 72*

7. To come out of this stretching posture straighten your elbows and in the same slow motion slide your hands up your legs until you are sitting in an upright position once again. Your head should be the last part of your body to straighten up.

8. Rest for a few moments and repeat the posture in exactly the same manner.

### Benefits to you

1. *The Complete Leg and Back Stretch* gives complete elasticity to the spine in the forward bending direction.

2. It removes deep tension throughout the spine and back.

3. The stretching out of the spine and subsequent relief from tension is one of the most marvelous therapeutic manipulations you can do for the health of your entire nervous system.

114

4. *The Complete Leg and Back Stretch* develops and tones the muscles of the back.

5. This exercise produces the ultimate elasticity of the legs, stretching the great gastrocnemius tendons behind the knees to their original natural flexibility.

6. It strengthens the legs.

7. The vertebrae of the spinal column are adjusted.

8. It helps reduce weight in the hips, abdomen and buttocks.

### Practice schedule

Do *The Complete Leg and Back Stretch* 3 times at each session. Hold it motionless for 10 seconds during the first week.

Add 5 seconds each week until you are holding it for 45 seconds. At this point you can perform the exercise only twice if you continue to add 5 seconds each week until you build your holding time up to one minute.

### Special hints

Although you will usually need considerable time before you can get into the complete position as shown in Fig. 71, the benefits to your body occur from the very first time that you practice the exercise.

Two main points are important for you to remember while performing *The Complete Leg and Back Stretch*:

1. Keep your legs straight at the knees. Every time you bend them you are cheating yourself out of time and results.

2. Do not fidget or adjust yourself once you are holding the stretch. You retard your progress by doing so. As in all the Yoga stretches hold it absolutely motionless in order to attain the full results.

When your hands come to be close to your ankles in the holding of this posture, you can bend your toes back toward you in an attempt to grasp them with your fingers.

## Exercise 20: THE BOW

MARVELOUS FOR DEVELOPING PERFECT POS-TURE AND STRENGTHENING THE LOWER BACK MUSCLES.

### How to practice this exercise

1. Lie on your mat on your abdomen with your hands at your sides. Let your body become completely limp (Fig. 73).

2. Turn your face so that your forehead is resting against the mat. Bring your toes and heels together (Fig. 74).

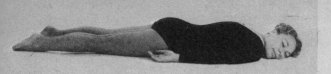

Figure 73

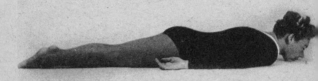

Figure 74

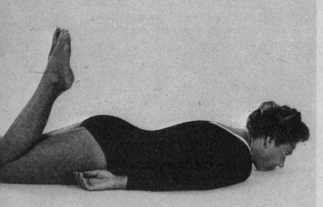

Figure 75

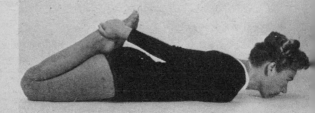

Figure 76

3. Bend both legs at the knees bringing your feet as close to your buttocks as you can (Fig. 75).

4. Reach back with your hands and grasp each foot with your respective hand (Fig. 76).

NOTE: If you are not able to grasp both feet with your hands, you should attempt to grasp one of them first and then the other, even if you have to shift to your side and manipulate your body in order to do so. Never under any circumstances, however, exert yourself strenuously. If you cannot grasp both feet at all with a moderate attempt, then simply grasp one foot with one hand and perform *The Bow* in that way alternating the feet each time until you gain enough strength and limberness to grasp both of them.

5. Raise your knees and thighs off the floor while at the same time you raise your head and trunk from the floor. Help yourself to perform this lifting movement by pulling your arms and legs against each other. Keep your head up and back as far as you can throughout the holding of the posture (Fig. 77).

6. Hold *The Bow* for 3 seconds. Breathe normally.

7. Lower yourself slowly out of *The Bow* posture by allowing your legs to come down first and then your trunk and head. Do this in a slow and controlled manner.

8. Release your legs and allow them to straighten out so that you are lying stretched out once again.

9. Go completely limp and rest for a few moments before you repeat the exercise.

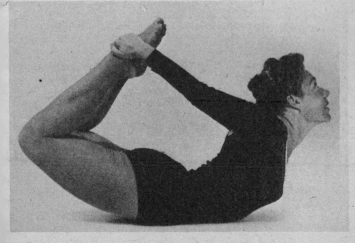

*Figure 77*

### Benefits to you

1. *The Bow* relieves tension throughout the entire back.
2. It adjusts the sacroiliac and lumbar vertebrae.
3. It is marvelous for the posture and has the ability to correct many serious postural faults.
4. It strengthens, firms and reduces the abdominal muscles.
5. It reduces weight in the hips and tightens the buttocks.
6. It strengthens the muscles of the arms and the thighs.
7. *The Bow* firms the muscles relating to the bust.
8. It develops the chest into beautiful lines.

### Practice schedule

Repeat *The Bow* 3 times at each workout.
Hold it motionless during the first week for 3 seconds.
Add 3 seconds each week until you are holding it for 15 seconds.

### Special hints

Remember the instructions relating to persons who cannot grasp both feet in the beginning. Manipulate your body, gently and carefully of course, however you must in order to grasp them.

The body has to adapt to the posture. This usually takes from one to three weeks if you practice regularly and correctly. Raise yourself up only as far as you can even if it involves only raising your legs off the ground and arching your head back. Your strength will develop in time as will your flexibility. Always move slowly and never strain under any circumstance.

Always hold your head back as far as you can. When going into the lift, keep your eyes up in their sockets. This will help you very much in holding the posture at the highest point.

In the beginning, if you feel that it is necessary, you can allow your knees to spread apart as you go up into *The Bow*. After a while, when your body has become somewhat accustomed to the exercise, you should try to keep your knees together. Keeping your knees together increases the effectiveness of the posture.

# CHAPTER SEVENTEEN

# Beauty and Health
# Through Good Posture

*About Posture*

The atrocities committed every day and all day against correct posture are staggering to contemplate. First, we attack and apparently attempt to destroy good posture by the way we sit and what we sit upon. Modern furniture runs high among the factors that tend to damage good posture. Usually the best chair we sit in each day, posture- and health-wise, is the relatively straight backed dining room chair. As for the others we flop into them and remain in them for extended periods of time in positions that could do no more to destroy the proper stance and carriage of our bodies than if we were trying to do so on purpose. Even when we sit in a chair in which we can maintain a normal, healthy, upright position, we usually slump forward in it so that we are resting on the base of the spinal column instead of on the buttocks with our bodies twisted to one side or another and our shoulders rounded.

In lying down—and this includes sleep—we are no better off. A great number of us sleep on mattresses that are too soft for the human body and which subject the spinal column to unnatural twists and positions that weaken various muscles and produce extremely bad effects upon our posture.

In standing, how many of us stand erectly with our weight distributed evenly on both legs. Most of the time we stand on one leg with the other somewhat limper and with all our weight upon one hip. In driving a car we slump into the soft seat. When at work or at school sitting at a desk, we further contribute to the deterioration of our natural healthy and esthetic carriage.

## Posture—A Major Key to Beauty

Posture is a major key to beauty. It is, to a great extent, our bearing and makes up for a multitude of imperfections in other areas of our appearance.

What is bad posture and how does it look to others? It is round shoulders. It is the suggestion of a hump in the upper middle portion of the spine. It is a sway back or the buttocks extended forward as if following the direction of a protruding abdomen. It is one shoulder higher than the other. It is hips out of line, or the appearance of excessive softness and weakness, of not caring how one looks. It is unsightly and ugly to the extreme.

Good posture on the other hand makes a person feel and look vital and fully alert to the life around them. It is chest held high as if the individual has some pride in herself. It is shoulders relaxed but properly placed and the lovely natural curve of the back and spine. It is the person looking healthful and alive. Your posture often reflects your general psychological outlook on life. Good posture works wonders for you. It improves your appearance, brings out your beauty, raises your morale and gives you confidence.

You have probably observed that nearly all the Yoga exercises you have learned so far have a definite beneficial effect upon your posture. You will find this to be the same with most of the Yoga exercises that are to follow. You can see how the *Backward Bend on the Toes, The Standing Twist, The Alternate Leg Pull, The Forehead to Heel Stretch, The Half Locust, The Plough,* and *The Twist,* to name a few of the exercises you have already learned, deal directly with posture and have a positive effect upon it.

The technique you will learn in this section, *The Backward Hand Clasp,* is a Yoga exercise which specifically affects that key area between and around the shoulder blades. This area is often the first to go if your posture deteriorates to the point where your spine and bearing are noticeably affected.

Besides the practice of these exercises, which are essential to your having lifelong good posture, I recommend that you walk correctly at all times, holding your head up high as if you were attempting to stretch your neck. Keep your chest up and, without straining in an unnatural fashion, try to bring your shoulder blades together as you walk. Do not carry this to the extreme extent of walking about in a ramrod manner. A good general rule for correct posture while walking or sitting (with your head and chest held high as indicated) has been stated in an earlier section. It consists of keeping your ears directly above your shoulders and your nose above your navel. If you can remember this clever little rule, you will enjoy the delight of correct posture and bodily carriage.

## Exercise 21: THE BACKWARD HAND CLASP

IMPARTS CORRECT POSTURE REACHING SELDOM USED MUSCLES RELATING TO THE SHOULDER BLADES.

### *How to practice this exercise*

1. This exercise can be practiced while standing or while sitting in a chair or in a cross-legged sitting position on the floor. I recommend that for purposes of formal practices you do it while seated in *The Half Lotus* position.

2. Raise your right arm directly into the air. Bend it at the elbow so that your right hand touches the center of your back. Your elbow is pointing straight up into the air.

3. Place your left hand behind you and bend your elbow so that the back of your left hand is against your spine. Your left arm will be in the position known in wrestling as the hammer lock (Fig. 78).

4. By carefully working your right hand down and at the same time inching your left hand upward, attempt to make your hands meet so that the fingers of each hand can clasp each other as in Fig. 79.

5. Hold this position motionless for 10 seconds.

6. Release your clasped fingers and come slowly out of the posture by reversing the steps in which you went into it.

7. Repeat the exercise, only reversing your hands so that your right arm will be behind your back and your left arm up in the air.

### *Benefits to you*

1. The main effect is a wonderful adjustment and training of your spine and back muscles so that you will gain the habit of perfect posture.

2. Seldom exercised muscles around and under your shoulder blades are developed.

3. Tight shoulder muscles are loosened.

4. The upper arms become firm.

### *Practice schedule*

Do *The Backward Hand Clasp* 3 times on each side, alternating your arms each time.

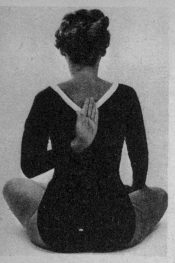
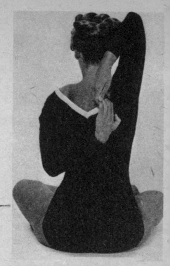

Figure 78                                        Figure 79

Hold your final position motionless for 10 seconds during the first week.

Add 5 seconds each week until you are holding it for 30 seconds.

### Special hints

This is an exercise that you can perform at any time during the day. It perks you up, gives a lift to your posture and relieves tension in the center of your back and in your shoulders.

Remember to move slowly making your hands creep inch by inch toward each other with your fingers.

The more upright you keep your upraised arm the better will be the results.

# CHAPTER EIGHTEEN

# Beauty and Health
# Through a Youthfully
# Limber Spine

## About the Spinal Column

The spinal column is a key area in the rebuilding and development of general health and beauty. The factor that makes the spinal column so essential to health is its relationship to the entire nervous system. From the brain there extends a long thin column of nerve tissue called the spinal cord. An extension of the brain itself, this delicate cord is encased in a protective sheath of bones we call the spinal column. The spinal column is composed of a number of separate bones called vertebrae. The vertebrae are separated from each other by a thin pad or disk.

The fact that the spinal column is composed of separate bones connected by ligaments enables the entire trunk of the body from the base of the spine to the neck to be flexible and to move in all different directions. Each of the vertebrae has openings to enable further extensions of the spinal cord to emerge from their column of protective bony armor and spread to every part of the body. These are the nerves. Thus we see that the nerves themselves are extensions of the brain. They are in a sense the brain itself having taken the form of the organism in order to function directly and perfectly with its environment.

## Spinal Column Must Be Pliable and Flexible

The spinal column was meant to be pliable and to be able to move freely in nearly every direction. The healthful condition of every part of the body is related to the ability of this column of connected bones to be moved and manipulated correctly. You see here, in simplified form, the basis of the science of chiropractic. This science is based on the knowledge that as the spinal column itself deteriorates and loses its natural flexibility and shape, every part of the body is negatively affected. Chiropractors then reverse the situation and remove the negative symptoms by correcting the improper spinal condition. Many a chiropractor who has attended my classes or lectures has told me in as few words that if everybody in the United States practiced Hatha Yoga every day there would not be a chiropractor left in business.

I recommend and extol all sports and exercises because they are all good for you. However, as far as scientifically reaching, manipulating, and developing every key area of the body, it is obvious now that sports accomplish only a fraction of the desired and necessary results. *Yoga is, in fact, the only complete science designed to help the individual to bring the spine back to its original natural condition and keep it that way.* That condition is one of great flexibility and elasticity.

The spinal column is contracted and stiffened prematurely in nearly all human beings. The reason for this is threefold.

1. The many unnatural factors of modern civilization.
2. Improper use of the spinal column through lack of knowledge of how it should be treated.
3. Simple lack of use.

Until someone has practiced Yoga for a while and has experienced its results, he cannot realize how badly contracted and stiffened the spine has become for the average person. When you practice Yoga for a few months, the limberness of your spinal column will have begun to be restored considerably and if you compare your flexibility with what it was when you first began the study of Yoga you will be amazed at the extent of the stiffening of the human body.

You have seen in the techniques which you have learned so far how Yoga treats the spine. It bends the spine in a methodical manner, which means in slow motion and holding the farthest position without moving, so that the body can stretch itself with complete relaxation. Yoga stretches the spine forward as in *The Alternate Leg Pull,* backward as in, for example, *The Bow,* in a spiral direction as in *The Twist,* and to the sides as in *The Side Bend.* The immediate results of performing these movements is the restoring of natural youthful flexibility to the spine and a profound relief from tension.

## Your Tensions Are Robbing You

Tension is the great robber of the enjoyment of living for modern people and nothing can so efficiently overcome this scourge as Yoga. Why do the stretching techniques of Yoga remove tension? It is simply because they reverse the way in which tension got there in the first place. When a human being is subjected to those influences, whether mental or physical, which cause tension, the body tightens up. This tightening of the muscles tends to become a habit as the tension producing experiences continue to press relentlessly upon the individual. The muscles, becoming tight, lose their pliability and cannot function completely. You have now removed the need for the tendons and ligaments to function completely since they are not called upon to do so. Add to this situation the general lack of use of our body in our modern time. The muscles and ligaments not being used, the joints become stiff in turn.

What Yoga does is simply to sit the body down and stretch the muscles out once again. Tendons and ligaments are stretched back to their normal resiliency resulting in the joints being able to move fully. It is normal and healthful for muscles and tissues to be highly flexible. The reason that many people experience "pulled" muscles or strained ligaments is because those tissues do not have the normal pliability that they are supposed to have. Thus, when pressure is put upon them, instead of giving like rubber, they tear.

Looking more deeply into the results of normal spinal flexibility, when the body is stretched the tension is relieved. When the tension is relieved the normal ability to relax is regained. When true relaxation occurs, your natural energy of life-force is able to function normally through your organism. A new vitality is experienced as a result of these exercises. Thus we see the relationship of relaxation to energy. Tension robs you of your natural vitality and Yoga, relieving that condition by the stretching method just described, enables you to live to your full capacity rather than to struggle along on one cylinder as most people do, wondering why there is no joy in living.

## Yoga Awakes Body and Mind

There is yet another and immensely profound result of the Yoga stretching postures. This has to do with the *awakening* of body and mind. There are powerful forces lying dormant—asleep—in each of our bodies. In our bodies there are certain centers at which these dormant forces tend to reside. One of these centers is the area of the spine. By practicing the Yoga exercises in the correct manner and with the correct state of mind, these dormant forces are awakened. When this occurs, the student experiences a true resurgence of life, vitality, awareness and expansion of consciousness. Here is the original purpose for the practice of Yoga many thousands of years ago. It is related to real peace of mind and spirit and to one's completion as a person.

A further word about flexibility of the spine. In the heading of this section I have used the expression "Beauty and Health Through a Limber Spine." A limber spine is the characteristic of youth, just as a stiff spine and body is the primary characteristic of age. When you attain flexibility of the spine by means of Yoga, you will, with the expenditure of a delightful few minutes a day, be able to keep your spine completely limber and flexible along with the rest of your body for the remainder of your life no matter how long you live. You will have all the results that come with the quality of elasticity, including strength, endurance and a strong, calm nervous system. You can prevent many aches, pains and even illnesses which are associated with the stiffening of the body. And, you will maintain the appearance and air of beauty that comes with a natural condition.

## Easy Does It in Yoga

You understand at this point how futile it is to attempt to force the body into a condition of flexibility. These exercises must be performed in a gentle manner. The entire system of Yoga is based on gentleness. In Yoga you learn the strength and power of gentleness. There are mental effects of these postures which correspond to the physical. You find as you practice that your outlook and your way of reacting to the world around you and to life becomes easier, gentler and softer. Rather than this gentle relaxed nature making you vulnerable to negative personalities or to the vicissitudes of life, you find that it, in itself, is a form of strength that overcomes the problems you have to face. Here is the beginning of serenity in the midst of the clashes, pressures and responsibilities of everyday living.

## Exercise 22: THE COBRA

STRETCHES EVERY VERTEBRA OF THE SPINAL
COLUMN TO ITS ORIGINAL NATURAL CONDITION
OF YOUTHFUL FLEXIBILITY.

### How to practice this exercise

1. Lie on your abdomen on your mat with your hands at your sides, palms up and your head resting on one cheek. Let your body become completely limp (Fig. 80).

2. Slowly turn your head so that it rests on your forehead (Fig. 81).

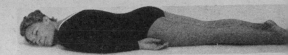

*Figure 80*

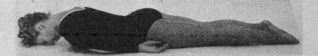

*Figure 81*

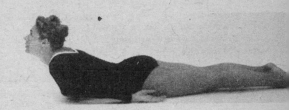

*Figure 82*

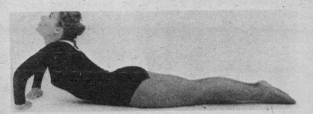

*Figure 83*

*Figure 84*

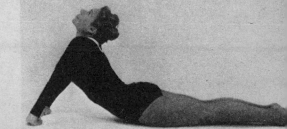

3. Very slowly raise your eyes to the top of their sockets. When they can go no further, slowly raise your head and back.

4. When your head can rise no further, continue raising your trunk up off the mat with the top of your chest leaving the floor first.

5. Raise your trunk in this manner, with your head back and your eyes up as far as they can look, until you can lift your trunk no further by the use of your back muscles alone (Fig. 82).

6. At this point, bring your arms slowly forward and place your hands, with your fingers pointing toward each other approximately six inches apart, under your chin (Fig. 83).

7. From this position, aided only slightly by your arms, continue to raise your trunk bending your spine upward and back until you can go no further comfortably. You should not allow your groin to be raised from the mat (Fig. 84).

8. When you have reached your limit of flexibility, hold your position motionless for the count of 10.

9. Begin coming down out of *The Cobra* posture by bending your arms slowly at the elbows and allowing your trunk to descend one inch at a time. First your stomach will touch the mat, then your middle chest, then your upper chest. Your head remains up and back until your entire chest is resting comfortably on the ground.

10. When you can support your upper body without the use of your arms, bring your arms slowly back to their original position at your sides.

11. Lower your head slowly and then your eyes until your forehead once more rests upon the mat.

12. Turn your face onto your cheek and go completely limp. Rest for several moments before repeating the exercise.

### Benefits to you

1. *The Cobra* manipulates, stretches and adjusts every vertebra of the spinal column from the neck to the base of the spine.

2. Youthful limberness is restored to the entire back and spine.

3. All the muscles, tendons and ligaments of the back are relaxed and relieved from tension.

4. *The Cobra* has a wonderful ability to dispel fatigue and it is especially good to perform when you arrive home from work.

5. The entire body is revitalized.

6. Posture improves.

7. The muscles of the chest and the bust are developed.

8. Back muscles are strengthened.

9. It firms and helps reduce the buttocks.

### Practice schedule

Do *The Cobra* 3 times at each session.

Hold it for 10 seconds during the first week.

Add 5 seconds each week, until you are holding it for 30 seconds each time.

If you tend to favor *The Cobra* posture you may feel free, if your time limitations permit, to continue increasing the holding time to 45 seconds.

### Special hints

You will feel the effects of this exercise immediately. *The Cobra* is another Yoga exercise that progresses very quickly. Your flexibility noticeably increases within a very few weeks.

It is absolutely essential to move in the proper slow motion in this exercise. It should take you at least 20 seconds to rise up into *The Cobra*. It is advisable for you to take 10 seconds simply to reach the point where you bring your arms forward. Slow motion is the key to success in Yoga. The slower you move when performing your postures, and the more absolutely motionless you hold your postures, the faster and deeper will be the results.

## Watch the Eyes

You have noticed the instructions about keeping your eyes focused up toward the top of your eye sockets. This is very important. You should conceive of the exercise as being led by the eyes. Imagine that a string is attached to each eyeball. The string is pulled up and back as if drawing your eyes up and then back toward your feet. When your eyes are drawn up, your head naturally follows in a backward direction thus raising the vertebrae in the region of your neck. The first vertebra bends upward and back. When the flexibility of the ligaments and tissue between and around the first and second vertebrae have reached their limit, the second vertebra will be drawn up and back by the first. The second will raise the third up and back which will raise the fourth and so on until each vertebra has followed the lead of your eyes and been raised individually. It is a curling motion rather than a bending at the waist. You should come down in the same way allowing one vertebra at a time to come to rest on the mat beginning with the lowest vertebra of your spine.

## This Is No Pushup

As you see, this is the farthest thing in the world from the pushup. Your groin does not leave the ground. If you find that your pelvis and thighs are rising off the floor, it means that your hands are down too close towards your chest. The arms are an adjusting lever in the exercise. The farther up toward your head that your hands rest on the floor, the easier the stretch will be for you. The farther down toward your chest that your hands rest, the more intense and difficult the stretch. Thus if you are particularly stiff in the beginning, I recommend that you place your hands on the floor up toward where your forehead rests.

Another important point about *The Cobra* concerns your heels. You will find that there is a tendency for your feet to spread apart in the beginning enabling you to have a greater stretch and to go up higher. It is a false flexibility, however, which will only cheat you out of the true limberness that you need. Keep your heels together throughout *The Cobra* posture. This is a basic rule for the correct performance of the exercise. It will make the stretch a bit more difficult, but you will be doing it correctly and in the long run you will be rewarded amply for your extra effort.

Proceed carefully if you are unusually stiff. Go up only as far as you can without undue strain or discomfort. If you are extremely stiff, I recommend that for the first week you do not stretch to your limit but go up only part way.

## Exercise 23: THE CHEST EXPANSION POSTURE

DEVELOPS THE CHEST AND FIRMS THE MUSCLES
THAT SUPPORT THE BUST FOR YOUTHFUL
LINES.

### How to practice this exercise

1. Stand erectly with your hands at your sides and your heels several inches apart (Fig. 85).
2. Raise your arms slowly up in front of you, elbows straight, so that your hands are touching each other at shoulder level, with the palms down (Fig. 86).
3. Slowly, with your elbows straight, bring your arms back around behind you at shoulder level as if doing the breast stroke in swimming.
4. When your arms can go no farther back, clasp your hands behind you by lowering your arms slightly or by bending your elbows.
5. When your hands are clasped, straighten both arms out behind you as high as you are able (Fig. 87).
6. Keeping your eyes open throughout, bend slowly back at the waist. Keep your knees straight. Let your head drop back with your neck limp so that you are looking upward at the ceiling. Bend back only as far as is comfortable (Fig. 88).
7. Hold the position motionless for 5 seconds.
8. Keeping your elbows straight and your hands firmly clasped behind you, straighten up slowly and without stopping bend slowly forward

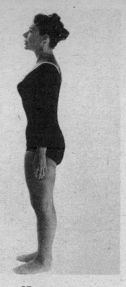

Figure 85

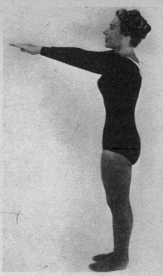

Figure 86

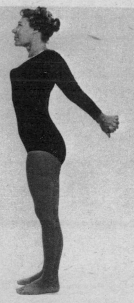

Figure 87

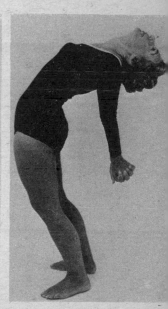

Figure 88

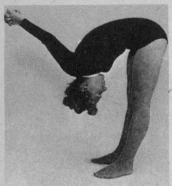

Figure 89

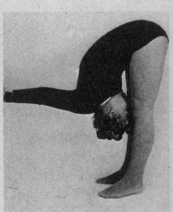

Figure 90

at the waist (Fig. 89) until your head is as far down toward the floor as you can comfortably reach. Your knees are straight. Your neck is limp. Make sure that you extend your arms forward as far as you can, as if trying to bring them over your head. Your ultimate aim is to have your forehead reach your knees (Fig. 90).

9. Hold the position motionless for 10 seconds.

10. Slowly straighten up until you are standing erectly.

11. Release your hands and allow your arms to come to rest at your sides.

12. Relax in this standing position for several moments and then repeat the same exercise.

### Benefits to you

1. The *Chest Expansion Posture* develops the chest and firms the muscles relating to the bust.

2. It is marvelous for improving the posture.

3. Flexibility of the spine in both backward and forward directions is promoted.

4. Tension throughout the entire body is relieved.

5. It is splendid for trimming and firming a flabby abdomen.

6. It improves the circulation of blood throughout the head which is beneficial for all the glands and organs of the head.

7. Seldom-used muscles of the shoulders are worked out.

### Practice schedule

During the first week of practicing the *Chest Expansion* hold the backward bending portion of it for 5 seconds and hold the forward bending portion of it for 10 seconds.

Add 5 seconds a week to the holding time of each of these positions.

Stop adding time to the backward bending position when you are holding it for 10 seconds. Add 5 seconds each week to the holding time of your forward bending position until you are holding it for 30 seconds.

Repeat the exercise 3 times.

### Special hints

Slow motion is of special importance in this exercise. You should take at least 5 seconds to go back into the backward stretch and you should take at least 15 seconds to go all the way forward into the forward stretching position. This is a particularly lovely and graceful movement and you should keep that in mind when practicing it. The more you realize the esthetic grace and loveliness of the Yoga postures as you perform them, the more benefits, physically and mentally, you will receive from them. It is important throughout the *Chest Expansion* posture to keep your arms up as high in back of you as you can in order to increase your benefits. Your arms are used as a lever here to control the pressure of your stretch. The more you press your arms toward your head in the forward position, the more intense your stretch will be.

Be careful when you bend backward. If you close your eyes you are liable to lose your balance.

The *Chest Expansion* posture is an amazingly quick reliever of tension throughout the body and it can provide you with a much needed quick lift during the day. I strongly advise you to find a place to be alone at some time during the workday, or whenever pressure is upon you, and perform 2 or 3 of the *Chest Expansion* postures. You will find it to be many times more refreshing, relaxing and energizing than several cups of coffee.

# CHAPTER NINETEEN

# Beauty and Health
for the Neck

*About the Neck*

The neck is a very delicate portion of the human anatomy and a universally recognized center of tension. The phrase "a pain in the neck" is a part of our everyday vocabulary. The neck, collecting neuro-muscular tension as it does, is subject to stiffness, pain and cramps of all sorts.

The fast moving or vigorous neck exercises with which many of us are familiar, do very little if anything to relieve tension in that area. If a person is older or has a particularly stiff neck, the customary fast exercises for the neck can even present a slight hazard.

Only slow and very gentle exercises are of any deep value. The following Yoga techniques are exceptionally soothing for the neck since they are so scientifically methodical and extremely gentle.

The neck has always been considered by artists and connoisseurs to be one of the key areas of beauty in the human body. The loveliness and esthetic qualities of your neck can be brought out if your neck is free from tension and when the muscles are strong, toned and relaxed.

### Exercise 24: THE NECK STRETCH

REMOVE TENSION AND ITS LINES FROM THE
NECK AS IF BY MAGIC.

### How to practice this exercise

1. This exercise is best practiced immediately after performing *The Cobra* posture. Begin by lying on your abdomen as you would be upon finishing *The Cobra*.

2. Prop yourself on your elbows and place your head in your cupped hands as shown in Fig. 91.

3. Turn your head to the left in such a manner that your chin rests in your left hand and the back of your head rests upon your right hand as shown in Fig. 92.

4. Now slowly turn your head as far as it can go without any unnatural strain and, with only the most gentle help of your hands, move your neck around to the left to its farthest comfortable limit.

5. Hold this stretch motionless for 5 seconds.

6. Now turn your head very slowly to the right until your chin is tucked in your right hand and the back of your head rests upon your left hand (Fig. 93).

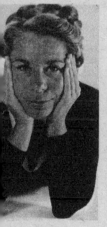

*Figure 91*

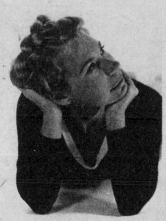

*Figure 92*

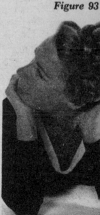

*Figure 93*

7. Perform the exact same stretch moving around toward your right.
8. Hold this stretch for 5 seconds.
9. Turn your head slowly toward the left again to repeat the exercise.

### Benefits to you

1. Tension in the neck is relieved no matter how deeply it has come to settle there.
2. It loosens and limbers a stiff neck.
3. The entire body relaxes.
4. Pain in the neck is relieved.
5. It irons out tension lines.

### Practice schedule

Perform *The Neck Stretches* 3 times on each side alternating from left to right to left, etc.

Hold your farthest position motionless for 5 seconds.

Add 5 seconds each week until you are holding it for 20 seconds.

### Special hints

Only slow motion scientific movements can truly remove tension and its discomforts from the area of the neck. It is quite important for you to move very gently and very carefully in this exercise. Make no sudden or strenuous movements while performing *The Neck Stretches*.

The correct hand and arm position is important here. Keep your elbows somewhat close as shown in the photographs so that your head will have the proper height. Do not raise your elbows off the mat at any time during the exercise.

If you keep your eyes closed while you are doing *The Neck Stretches*, you will experience a most delightful, relaxing sensation.

The exercise can be performed while sitting if you prop your elbows on a table. For a quick relief from a tension-induced minor ache in your neck during the day, you can perform a variation of this stretch without resting your elbows upon any surface. It is far better, however, to do the exercise in the manner instructed with your elbows propped upon a surface.

---

## NECK EXERCISE VARIATIONS

FOR RELIEF FROM TENSION IN THE NECK.

### The Slow Neck Roll

1. Drop your head very slowly until your neck is completely limp and your head hangs forward onto your chest (Fig. 94).

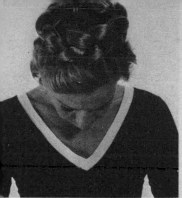

Figure 94

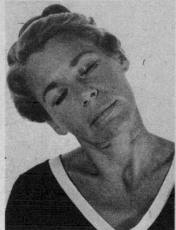

Figure 95

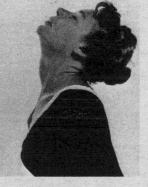

Figure 96

2. Very slowly roll your head around to your right side. Keep your neck limp and let the weight of your head pull your neck muscles (Fig. 95).

3. Continue moving your head very slowly around until it is hanging back (Fig. 96) and then continue around toward your left and finally back to your forward beginning position.

4. Perform the same movement rolling your head around to your left.

5. Do the *Slow Neck Roll* 3 times alternating the direction each time from right to left.

6. It should take you 30 seconds to perform each roll of your head.

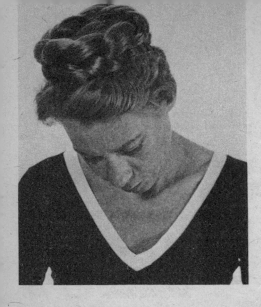

*Figure 97*

### The Slow Neck Drop

INDUCES DEEP RELAXATION THROUGHOUT THE
ENTIRE BODY.

1. Sit erectly in a chair, your feet flat upon the floor, your hands resting limply, palms up on each thigh. Do not let your hands touch each other.

2. Lower your eyelids but do not close your eyes.

3. Let your lips part and become loose and limp. Let your lower jaw relax and drop slowly so that your teeth are apart.

4. Moving slowly, taking at least 1 full minute to do so, let your head fall slowly forward, slightly to one side—just a little off center—until your head is hanging limply in the position indicated in Fig. 97 and your chin is against or underneath your collar bone.

5. By the time you have lowered your head all the way as shown in Fig. 97 you should have closed your eyes.

6. You will find this exercise to be so utterly relaxing that you may feel like going directly to sleep. The exercise is marvelous to practice immediately before going to sleep at night. When the lights are out and you are about to retire, perform this movement while sitting up in bed. It brings about the most wonderful relaxation and quick sleep.

Both of these variations can be done after *The Neck Stretches,* as part of your regular Yoga workout, and also at any time during the day when needed.

# CHAPTER TWENTY

# Beauty and Health
for the Face

*About the Face*

Tens of millions of dollars are spent by women every year for lipstick, powder, rouge, mascara, eyebrow pencil, eye shadow, eye liner, night cream, under eye cream, powder base, astringent, facial pack, dry skin cream, beauty grains for skin peeling, deep pore cleanser, cleansing creams for make up removal, vanishing cream, moisturizer, skin activators and numerous other cosmetics.

*What Do Cosmetics Really Do?*

What is the purpose of all of this expense and care? It is to create beauty. But let us ask the question in the following manner. *What do these cosmetics actually do?* We are aware that proper use of cosmetics can certainly enhance the appearance of a woman's face. Looking at it in a deeper esthetic sense, however, we must say that these products are used to create a mask, a substitute face, as it were.

Let us inquire further. What is the mask being used in place of? Is the mask of cosmetics really being used to bring out a woman's innate beauty or is it used as a substitute for a natural beauty that can no longer reveal itself?

The implication is that make up is applied to the face in direct proportion to the imperfections that have come to exist there. We see in every-day life how the application of make up ranges from a lovely subtle re-finement, such as a shade of tasteful lipstick and perhaps a touch of pencil to the eyebrows, or mascara to the lashes, to masks of outrageous vulgarity and horror.

The natural face—for which all this money, trouble and time is attempting to substitute—is a glowing complexion with the full natural color that a woman should have regardless of her skin type. It should be a clear and alert face, bright-eyed and free from lines of strain and tension.

The face more than any single physical part of the body is the mirror of the real nature of the individual. We have all seen faces that reflect negative conditions of our times: anxiety, worry and fear. We have seen faces reflect the evils in which people unfortunately become involved such as hate, envy, greed, and so forth. The face *should* reflect the great and noble attributes that are natural to the human spirit such as serenity, love, compassion, calm self-assurance, inner peace and tolerant understanding. The only *true* beauty that will ever be manifested by any person will be that beauty which reflects the inner nature or state of mind of that individual. Yoga, through its incredible power to alleviate mental and physical tension, removes those veils (anxiety, fear, worry, tensions, strain, fatigue) that hide the true nature and beauty of a person.

## *What Yoga Can Do for Your Face*

When the body is relieved of nervousness, tension, tightness, and stiffness, the mind is correspondingly relieved. The tranquility that human beings are supposed by nature to have can then at last shine forth. As time goes by and you practice your Yoga exercises regularly, you will hear people say to you, "You look so calm all the time," or "You look years younger."

The first technique that you will be taught in this section, *The Lion,* is an ingenious Yoga exercise which concentrates specifically on the face. It has been used by innumerable people for thousands of years to accomplish all the results that are claimed for it.

In combination with Yoga exercises that emphasize the improvement of circulation throughout the face, you should experience wonderful results in a short time from *The Lion*.

### Exercise 25: THE LION

STRETCHES AWAY TENSION LINES IN THE FACE.
HELPS PREVENT WRINKLING.

### *How to practice this exercise*

1. Sit in *The Japanese Sitting Position* as you have been previously instructed or in any other comfortable cross-legged sitting position. Your hands should rest palms down upon your thighs (Fig. 98).

2. Arch your back slightly forward. Stretch your arms out stiffly at the elbows. Spread your fingers far apart.

3. Open your mouth as wide as you can and at the same time open your eyes as wide as possible.

4. Extend your tongue out of your mouth as far as it will go as if attempting to touch the point of your chin with it (Fig. 99).

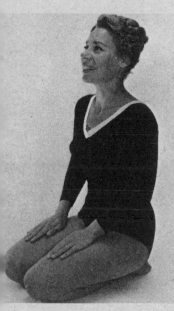

Figure 98

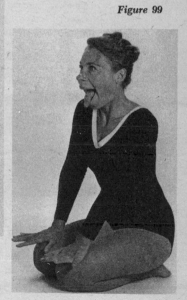

Figure 99

5. Hold this position motionless for 15 seconds.

6. Draw your tongue back into your mouth, close your mouth and relax your face completely. Allow your hands to relax limply upon your thighs and relieve the slight forward arching of your spine.

7. Sit for several moments enjoying the delightful sensation in your face as you feel the immediate relief from tension.

8. Repeat the exact same movement for the prescribed number of times.

## Benefits to you

1. *The Lion* tightens sagging face and neck muscles.

2. Tension throughout the entire face is relieved.

3. Certain lines of strain and fatigue are removed.

4. It helps remove a double chin.

5. It perks up the face, giving you a feeling of vibrancy and of being refreshed.

6. *The Lion* improves circulation throughout the face.

7. Circulation in the throat area is stimulated.

8. It tones the facial tissues and improves the complexion.

9. A great deal of premature wrinkling can be prevented and certain types of lines and wrinkles that already exist, especially around the corners of the eyes and the lips, can be eliminated.

10. The larynx is stimulated and massaged.

11. It has the ability to relieve sore throats.

12. It is beneficial for the salivary glands.

## Practice schedule

Repeat *The Lion* posture 3 times at each sitting.

Hold it for 15 seconds for the first week.

After the first week increase your holding time to 30 seconds and continue with that time from then on. *The Lion* posture is a technique that you can practice at any time throughout the day when you feel the need for it. It is wonderful for a quick relief of tension in face. If you wish to combat a facial problem with greater emphasis, you can do *The Lion* 3 times in succession several times a day, for example 3 times in the morning, 3 times in the afternoon and 3 times in the evening. You cannot overdo this exercise and you may feel free to perform it as many times as you wish.

## Special hints

*The Lion* posture as is evident at first sight is rather funny looking. I remember how in class I am accustomed to telling my students that they can make good use of odd moments during the day to gain the remarkable benefits of this exercise. I recommended that they could even perform it with slight modifications while driving in their automobiles. Sometime later one of my students told me how she had been riding in her car one quiet Sunday morning and had decided that this was a good occasion to perform *The Lion.* She opened her mouth wide and stuck her tongue way out as she drove along. Suddenly, she began to get a peculiar feeling and glancing to her side she saw four extremely dignified old ladies, who were obviously on their way home from church, riding in a car next to her and staring incredulously at her.

I would advise you to avoid having other people observe you doing this exercise. In the event, however, that anyone might ever laugh at you for practicing *The Lion,* I urge you to remember that you will have the last laugh as your face develops and retains the lovely glow of health.

As with all Yoga exercises, *The Lion* is a completely natural movement. Keep your eyes wide open throughout the exercise. The muscles around the eyes and the lips are circular and this is the only true tension relieving stretch they can receive.

### Exercise 26: THE COW

IMPROVES THE COMPLEXION BY INCREASING
CIRCULATION TO THE FACE.

#### How to practice this exercise

1. Stand erectly with your heels about three inches apart and your arms at your sides (Fig. 100).

2. Slowly raise your arms forward and up until they are straight in the air above your head (Fig. 101). As you raise your arms, which should take you at least 10 seconds, you should inhale a *Complete Breath*.

3. As soon as your arms are straight up over your head begin bending forward so that you can eventually attempt to reach your toes or farther with your hands. Exhale as you begin to bend forward.

NOTE: This movement does not consist simply of "bending at the waist." By bending at the waist you will be depriving most of your spine and back of the therapeutic effects of the stretch. The correct way to bend forward in *The Cow* is to begin moving your arms downward while making your head follow your arms as you lower them. Do this by keeping your ears directly between your arms, even touching them. This will make certain that the vertebrae and muscles of your neck stretch and bend forward first. When your head has bent forward between your arms until your chin is tucked against or near your jugular notch at the top of your breastbone (Fig. 102), then continue "curling" your spine down keeping

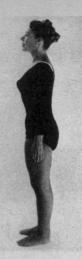

*Figure 100*

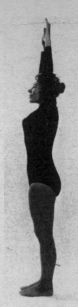

*Figure 101*

*Figure 102*

*Figure 103*

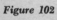

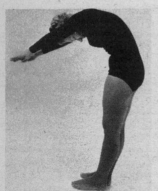

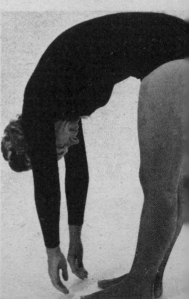

your face and arms close to your body until eventually your entire spine is bent forward down to your waist and lower back (Fig. 103). The curling method of bending your spine is basic to Yoga and you should keep it in mind as a model when performing any of the other forward or backward stretching exercises.

It should take you at least 20 seconds to bend all the way down from your upright position.

4. When your body cannot be bent farther forward by the weight of your trunk, in the same slow motion grasp your legs at whatever part you can comfortably reach (Fig. 104).

5. Bending your elbows, gently and very slowly pull yourself down to your farthest comfortable limit aiming your forehead toward your knees.

6. Hold this position for 10 seconds (Fig. 105).

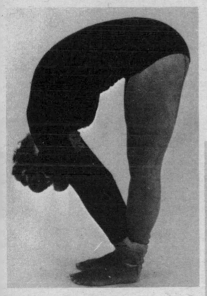

Figure 104

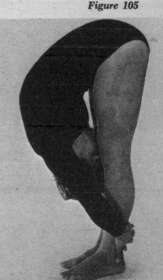

Figure 105

7. Come up by releasing your grip upon your legs and rising upright in exactly the reverse manner in which you went down. Remember to keep your head between your upper arms and to curl your spine up so that one vertebra is straightened at a time. Your head should be the last part of your body to become erect. When your arms are once more extended straight upward, bring them down slowly to your sides. It should take you as long to come up in the correct slow motion as it does to go down into the posture.

8. Stand in a relaxed manner for a few moments before repeating the exercise.

### Benefits to you

1. *The Cow* posture increases the circulation of blood throughout the head and face which improves the complexion. It is especially effective when practiced in conjunction with *The Lion* posture.

2. Tension is relieved from the entire spine and back and youthful elasticity is promoted.

3. The legs, especially the great tendons in the back of the legs, become flexible.

4. *The Cow* is splendid for relieving general physical tension and can be used many times during the work day for that reason.

5. It is relaxing and revitalizing for the entire body and excellent for overcoming fatigue.

### Practice schedule

Perform *The Cow* 3 times.
Hold your farthest position for 10 seconds during the first week.
Add 5 seconds each week until you are holding it for 30 seconds.

### Special hints

When you have gone down into *The Cow* posture, you should make sure before you grasp your legs that your entire trunk is hanging limply at the waist so that its full weight is pulling against the supporting muscles and tendons.

Bear in mind the two principles of Yoga stretching which are exemplified in *The Cow*. The first is that the sheer weight of one part of the body (in this instance the trunk) is enough to stretch the muscles and ligaments back to their natural pliability. The second principle is that gentle, steady pressure will stretch the body more efficiently and make it more flexible than most strenuous movements.

Remember to be motionless while holding the position. There is a temptation in *The Cow* posture to bob up and down slightly in order to

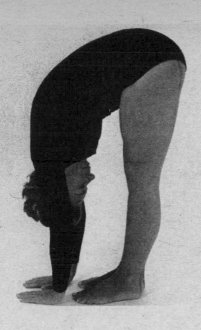

*Figure 106*

gain a greater stretch. Do not give in to this temptation. It will only detract from the wonderful results that you can obtain from the exercise.

You may find at first that you are quite stiff and that your hands can reach down only as far as your knees or slightly below them. In time, however, the gastrocnemius tendon behind your legs as well as your tension stiffened back and spine will relax and loosen and you will be able to perform *The Cow* posture by placing your hands upon the floor as in Fig. 106.

Breathe normally throughout the exercise.

# CHAPTER TWENTY-ONE

# Beauty and Health for the Eyes

## About the Eyes

The eyes are a much abused and much misunderstood organ of the body. The first thing to know is that all eye exercises must be done with the goal of relaxation in mind and thus in a relaxed way. The muscles of the eyes are subject to much tension and what is needed is not only a relaxed exercising of the eyes but also the habit of relaxed use of the eyes.

## The Effect of Your Eyes on Your Nervous System

What you do to your eyes, whether positive or negative, affects your entire nervous system. The more you can relax your eyes the more soothed and tranquil your nervous system will be. A good suggestion regarding the use of your eyes is to avoid staring fixedly at things. Always remember to keep your attention moving in a relaxed leisurely manner over the objects in the world around you. This applies to reading as well as general use.

The following exercises are designed to relax the eye muscles. The results of these exercises are reflected in clear eyes, a serene look, and the elimination of strain and underlying fatigue.

An excellent thing to do after you finish these exercises is to apply, on a washrag or a small towel, alternating applications of cold and warm water to your closed eyes. You will be absolutely delighted with the result of performing these exercises and then applying the cold and warm applications.

## Exercise 27: THE EYE MOVEMENTS

RELIEVE TENSION, HEADACHE AND EYE ACHE
THAT COMES FROM NERVOUS OR VISUAL STRAIN.

### *How to practice this exercise*

There are four procedures to *The Eye Movements*.

A.

(1) Sit in a relaxed manner either cross-legged on your mat or in *The Japanese Sitting Position*, whichever is the most comfortable for you. Your eyes will be open throughout the first exercise.

(2) Visualize in front of you a large clock with the numbers from 1 to 12 in bold letters situated on it as they are on an ordinary clock face.

(3) Look up at the imaginary number 12 on the top of the clock dial. Make sure that your eyes look as far as possible to the limit of their sockets when practicing this technique (Fig. 107).

(4) In a rhythmic staccato manner begin moving your eyes clockwise around the dial stopping for an instant at each imagined number. Hold your head straight forward and do not allow it to move. Only your eyes move (Fig. 108).

*Figure 107*    *Figure 108*

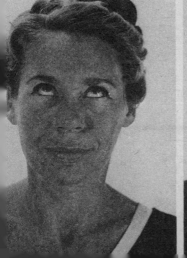 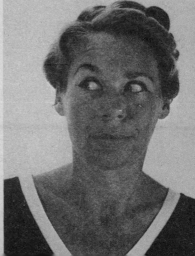

(5) When you have gone around the entire circle with your eyes and are back at number 12 on the top again, perform the exact same movement in the opposite direction or counterclockwise, moving from 12 to 11 to 10, etc.

(6) Perform the movement around in a complete circle 3 times, alternating from clockwise to counterclockwise.

(7) Close your eyes and rest for at least 30 seconds before performing the next movement.

B.

(1) The second eye movement is exactly the same as the first, except for two factors.

(a) It is performed with the eyes closed. You may even cup your hands over your eyes if you are in a particularly bright place. Do not, however, allow your palms to actually touch your eyes (Fig. 109).

(b) This movement is done in a more relaxed easy-going manner than the first. You should ease the stretch ever so slightly by not forcing your eyes to look to the very limit of their sockets.

(2) Perform the movement the same number of times as the first; that is 3 times around alternating the direction each time.

C.

(1) This movement has to be done in the outdoors or in front of a window.

(2) Hold your index finger up in front of your face about six inches away from your eyes. Focus your eyes upon the tip of your finger or upon your fingernail. Do not allow it to waver or gaze at anything else (Fig. 110).

*Figure 109*                                    *Figure 110*

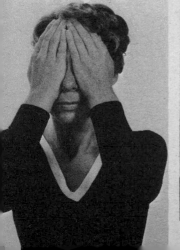
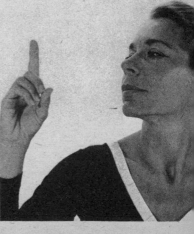

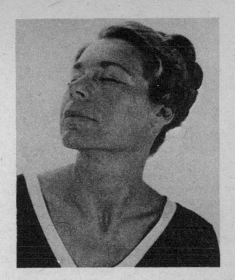

*Figure 111*

(3) After focusing your eyes upon your fingertip for approximately 3 seconds, quickly look at the most distant object available to you. It can be a distant tree, a cloud, or a hill. Make your eyes focus on that object as sharply and as clearly as possible and concentrate strongly on it.

(4) When you have focused your eyes upon the distant object for approximately 3 seconds, bring your eyes back as quickly as you can and focus them on the tip of your finger once again.

(5) Continue alternating from fingertip to very distant object 10 times in succession.

D.

(1) It is recommended that this fourth technique be practiced out of doors where you can use the sun. If, however, conditions are such that it is impractical to practice it outdoors, you should perform in front of a strong light bulb keeping the light bulb at approximately 6 to 9 inches from your eyes.

(2) We will presume that you are performing the technique outside using the sun. Sit comfortably in as relaxed a manner as you can. Close your eyes. Turn your head so that your eyes are facing the sun (Fig. 111).

(3) Letting the full power of the sun glare upon your lids and warm both your eyes, slowly roll your head from left to right and then back again. Do not move your eyes consciously or consciously focus them toward the sun. Simply move your head in this manner with the light and the warmth of the sun upon your lids.

151

(4) Move your head from left to right and then back to the left again 10 times very slowly keeping your neck, face and body as limp as possible.

(5) If the sun is too weak outside or if there is no sun at all or the weather is bad, do the same thing using a light bulb as instructed. This incidentally is a splendid technique to perform with a light bulb immediately before going to sleep for the night. It has a wonderful ability to relax the nervous system and induce deep restful sleep.

### Practice schedule

The practice schedule for *The Eye Movements* has been given in the instructions themselves.

It is advisable to practice them all in succession as one closely related series of exercises, or you can adapt the exercises to your own time limitations. If you cannot do them all together, you will receive the same benefit if you practice them at different times during the day.

### Benefits to you

1. *The Eye Movements* relieve tension in the eyes, making them young and beautiful.
2. They are deeply relaxing for the entire nervous system.
3. Eye fatigue is immediately relieved.
4. The eye muscles are strengthened.

### Special hints

These movements are splendid to perform when your eyes are tired and when your body is fatigued or tense from the day's activities and pressures.

When you are finished with *The Eye Movements,* lie down and let your body go entirely limp for at least a minute so that you can fully experience the relaxation that comes with the doing of these exercises.

# PART THREE

# Eight

# Major Exercises

# for Health

# and Beauty

# CHAPTER TWENTY-TWO

# The Supreme Exercise
# for Women

## About the Inversion Postures

We see now that Yoga is a system of passive exercises. Conscious manipulation of the body in Yoga is held to a physical minimum. What we strive for is simply to place the body in a certain position in order to allow the body itself to bring about certain results. In Yoga you are helping your body bring forth qualities that are innately and intrinsically yours already. The inversion postures of Yoga are perfect examples of passive exercise in which you yourself practice "being still and doing nothing" while nature brings about the most wonderful results. The two basic inversion postures are *The Shoulder Stand* and *The Head Stand*.

### Exercise 28: THE SHOULDER STAND

*The Shoulder Stand* is the first complete inversion posture that you will learn in this course. Inversion postures deal primarily with the improvement of circulation throughout the entire body. They are designed to affect the circulation in such a manner that excessive pressure is relieved from the veins and arteries of the legs and increased circulation is provided to the organs and glands of the upper part of the body.

*How to practice the shoulder stand*

1. Lie on your back on your mat with your hands at your sides. Let your body become completely limp (Fig. 112).

2. Bring your hands close to your sides and turn them so that your palms are facing down (Fig. 113).

3. Tighten your abdominal muscles and stiffen your legs. Aiding yourself by pressing downward against the floor with your hands, begin to lift your legs slowly off the floor. Keep your knees straight (Fig. 114).

4. Slowly raise your legs until they are straight up in the air at a ninety degree angle to your body. You should do this as slowly as you possibly can. The slower you can raise your legs the stronger you will make your abdomen (Fig. 115).

5. When you have reached this point, with an increased pressure of your hands against the floor and by using the muscular power of your abdomen and back, raise your buttocks and lower back off the floor as shown in Fig. 116. If you have difficulty in raising yourself in this manner, you may perform whatever rocking movements or efforts are necessary to get up into the position.

6. Place your left hand against the kidney region of your back and brace yourself with it (Fig. 117).

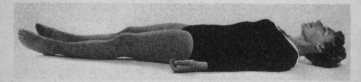

*Figure 112*

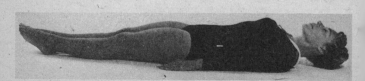

*Figure 113*

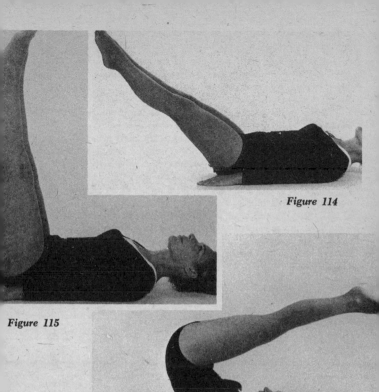

Figure 114

Figure 115

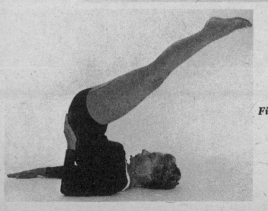

Figure 116

Figure 117

7. Place your other hand against your lower back for support (Fig. 118) and continue raising your body until you are in or as close as you can get to the complete position of *The Shoulder Stand* as shown in Fig. 119.

8. Hold the position motionless for the time indicated in the *Practice Schedule*.

9. To come down from the posture, first bend your legs at the knees until your knees are an inch or two above your face. Needless to say all movements are performed in slow motion (Fig. 120).

10. Place your right hand against the floor and brace yourself with it (Fig. 121). Then place your left hand on the floor. You are now in the position as shown in Fig. 122.

11. Keeping the back of your head against the floor at all times throughout the remainder of the exercise, and controlling the movement of your body with the pressure of your hands against the floor, roll slowly forward until your lower back rests again upon your mat (Figs. 123 and 124).

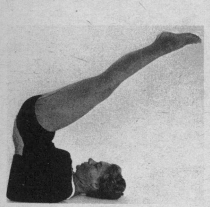

*Figure 118*

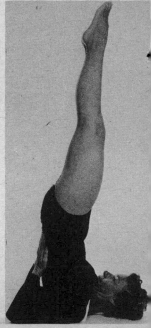

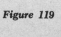

*Figure 119*

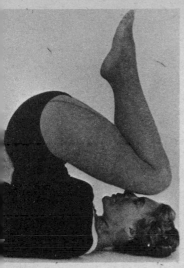

Figure 120

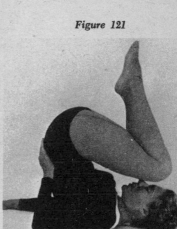

Figure 121

Figure 122

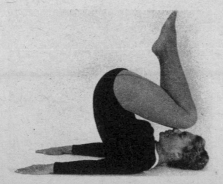

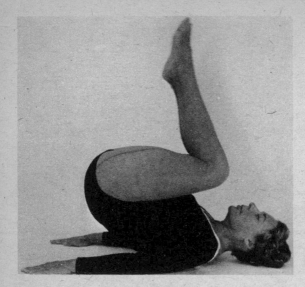

*Figure 123*

*Figure 124*

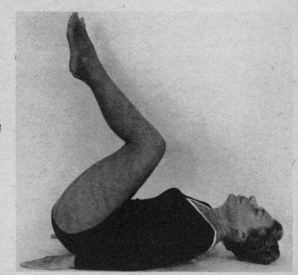

160

12. Slowly straighten your legs until they are once more directly vertical in the air.

13. Keeping your knees straight, lower your legs as slowly as you can until they are resting on the ground. Do not allow yourself to "give up" when you near the end of the lowering motion. Never collapse out of any Yoga postures but keep your discipline until the very end.

14. Once more allow your body to become completely limp from toes to head and rest for at least 2 minutes after coming out of *The Shoulder Stand*. You will feel the immediate effects of the posture by resting in this manner.

### Practice schedule

Begin by holding *The Shoulder Stand* for 1 minute during the first week.

Add 1 minute each week until you are standing in *The Shoulder Stand* for 3 minutes.

Three minutes is the minimum amount of time that it takes for *The Shoulder Stand* to do its work.

As long as you build your time up slowly and methodically at this rate, you may feel free to go beyond the 3 minute holding time and advance to 5 minutes.

### Benefits to you

The benefits of *The Shoulder Stand* to the human body are so numerous that it is scarcely conceivable that any one exercise can produce such deep and dynamic results. However, all the results claimed for *The Shoulder Stand* have been verified by experience and by research. I will enumerate these beneficial effects beginning with the legs and working toward the head.

1. When you place your body in *The Shoulder Stand, it is easier for the heart to pump blood through the blood vessels of the legs* enabling the veins in the legs to relax. They are freed temporarily from the continuous strain and *pressure that gravity imposes* upon them when the body is in its customary upright position. The strain upon the blood vessel walls being relieved, they have a chance to regenerate and regain their normal strength and condition. This Yoga posture has been found to greatly aid in relieving numerous cases of varicose veins.

2. Similarly gravity pulls downward upon the organs and glands of our body all the day long. When inverting the body in *The Shoulder Stand*, these *organs and glands fall back up into their proper positions,* especially the organs and glands in the viscera which tend to sag as the abdominal muscles weaken through the years. Besides the highly therapeutic replace-

ment of these vital organs and glands there is also a wonderful relaxing effect upon them. The organs and tissues from which they hang and upon which they rest are relieved by the reversal.

3. More and more doctors every year are recommending that women practice *The Shoulder Stand* after childbirth. *For post-childbirth use* of this posture, a woman should simply eliminate the lifting of the legs in the straight manner as instructed. If you are a woman who has just given birth, you can get into the posture by first bending your legs at the knees and making it as easy as you can to lift your lower back off the floor. The inverted position of *The Shoulder Stand* allows the organs and glands that are related to childbirth, and which have been under tremendous strain due to pregnancy and parturition, to fall back gently, effortlessly and very exactly into their proper place.

4. *The Shoulder Stand* is a *wholesome rejuvenator of the sexual glands and organs*. This is especially true of the male sex glands.

5. *The Shoulder Stand* has been known to aid in *relieving hemorrhoids*.

6. There is a *stimulation of circulation* throughout the *visceral organs*.

7. *The heart tends to rest* in this position due to the greater ease of pumping blood throughout the legs and to the upper part of the body.

8. Of all the effects of *The Shoulder Stand,* the most noteworthy is the effect upon the *body weight. The Shoulder Stand* has a very strong and direct influence upon regulating and normalizing your weight. In most instances it will *reduce weight*. In many instances of underweight it will help you add weight because of its effect upon the thyroid gland.

The thyroid gland is located in the region of the throat and is directly involved with increases or decreases of weight in the human body. It is a weight regulator. Due to faulty eating habits, lack of proper exercise and other factors, the thyroid gland does not function correctly in many people. It becomes sluggish and does not perform the function that is necessary to maintain normal body weight.

By inverting your body in *The Shoulder Stand* the blood, in increasing throughout the upper portion of your body, comes to pump directly and strongly through and around the thyroid gland. This increased circulation is aided by maintaining a correct neck position while in the posture which consists of keeping the chin snugly against the jugular notch as shown in the illustration of the complete position of this exercise. The increased circulation is an actual internal massage of the thyroid gland since it stimulates and regulates the gland so that it can function normally.

*The Shoulder Stand* is a wholesome natural technique for you to perform. You will be amazed and gratified at the results on your weight. The results are especially enhanced when you practice a complete daily schedule of Yoga exercises. A schedule specifically designed for people who wish to combat and overcome a weight problem is presented in the section entitled *Practice Schedules For Special Problems*.

9. *The Shoulder Stand* increases and *improves circulation throughout the entire upper part of the body*.

10. All the glands and organs of the head are benefited by increased circulation through them including the *eyes, ears, and salivary glands*.

11. The improved circulation in the head and face is splendid for the *complexion*.

12. Of great importance is the way in which *The Shoulder Stand directly affects the brain itself*. The increased (and it is a moderate increase) circulation throughout the upper body and head goes directly into all the blood vessels in the brain itself. The brain, due to the difficulty of circulating blood properly throughout the head during our everyday life is habitually starved for the nourishment which it is the task of the blood to bring to all the parts of the body. When circulation is thus improved in the brain, the student will find a new and delightful freedom from mental and nervous fatigue. The brain is stimulated and I have been told of cases of improvement of certain mental faculties such as the memory.

13. The increased circulation through the scalp and the hair roots is of benefit to the *hair*. Baldness itself is not hereditary. The only thing that is inherited is the tendency to become bald if certain negative environmental conditions are present. The strongest negative condition that can make a hereditary tendency toward baldness become an actuality is poor circulation in the scalp. I maintain that if a person has proper body circulation the chances of his becoming bald are enormously reduced.

14. We have followed the effects of *The Shoulder Stand* from the legs to the top of the head. As we can see, it has marvelous results upon the total body circulation. *The Shoulder Stand* also provides the body with *deep overall relaxation*. You will experience this immediately upon coming down out of it. Due to its effect upon the brain the entire nervous system is strengthened by the posture. Medical science has also recently verified the fact that *The Shoulder Stand* is of great aid in relieving asthmatic conditions.

### Special hints

I will never forget a statement one of my students made in class one day. We had reached *The Shoulder Stand* in the course and I had just placed them all into it for the first time. I wanted to give them time to experience what it is like to remain in the position for three minutes. Realizing that many of them were not used to such activity, I decided that now would be a good time to tell them about the effects *The Shoulder Stand* has upon reducing weight. I concluded my statements and looked at my watch. They still had another minute or so in which to stand there motionless. It occurred to me then that here was an opportunity to tell them of certain techniques they could use to overcome any restlessness they might feel while standing in this position for three minutes. In order to introduce the subject, I said,

"You may be unaccustomed to remaining motionless in this manner for even as small a time as three minutes. What do you think would be a practical and sensible activity to engage in while standing in *The Shoulder Stand?*"

From the back row there came the voice of an extremely stout woman who had struggled very hard to get up into *The Shoulder Stand* in her dedication to losing weight.

"We can eat something," she said.

I would not advise this as a practical course to follow. There are much better physical and mental activities you can engage in while in *The Shoulder Stand.*

One of them is *The Eye Movements* which you have learned. Being in *The Shoulder Stand* is a splendid time for you to do them since there is a healthful increase in circulation through those organs at this time.

The very fact that you will have to stand for the required number of minutes in the posture or that you must remain in the other Yoga stretching exercises for a certain amount of time in itself has a profoundly positive effect upon your mind as well as your body. We live in civilization characterized by "the pace that kills." Learning to remain motionless yet at the same time relaxed in these positions frees us from the unnatural neurotic hurry to which we have become accustomed. Later, in the section entitled *Beauty and Health Through Peace of Mind*, you will learn a mental exercise designated to promote tranquility and peace. You can practice that exercise (*Meditation Upon the Breath*) while in *The Shoulder Stand.*

Remember to go up into *The Shoulder Stand* only as far as you comfortably can. Never strain in an attempt to attain the completed posture. Your body will adapt to *The Shoulder Stand* very quickly and in a short time you will find yourself standing vertical in perfect posture.

If through *overweight, age, or excessive stiffness* you are unable to go into *The Shoulder Stand* at all in the beginning, you should do the following until you are able to raise and keep your lower back off the floor.

Simply lean your legs against a wall or against the back of a sturdy chair and allow that alteration in your circulation to take place. Every time you practice in this modified manner, attempt to raise your body a little more off the floor with the aid of your legs pressing against the wall or chair and your hands pushing upward against your lower back. In time the muscles of your abdomen and back will develop and with the increased strength and fitness that your other Yoga exercises bring, you will be able to get up into *The Shoulder Stand* and eventually go all the way in it.

If you feel a throbbing of blood in your face or throat while in *The Shoulder Stand*, that is a very good sign and you should welcome the sensation. It means that your head and face have been so starved for proper circulation that they are unused to the sensation of blood flowing through them. In a very few days the sensation will leave as your blood vessels and tissues become accustomed to the increased circulation.

Breathe normally throughout *The Shoulder Stand* and try to keep your body as relaxed as you can while holding the position. You are not supposed to keep your body rigidly erect. You are supposed to keep it erect in a relaxed fashion. Only your biceps should be tight during *The Shoulder Stand*.

You can, providing you do so in the proper slow motion, move your legs in certain ways while in the posture. You can allow them to spread apart—doing "the split"—with your knees straight while you are in this inverted position. You will be receiving the same circulatory benefits and you will be stretching the seldom used muscles and tendons on the insides of your legs from the groin through your knee area. You can also practice stretching your legs by spreading them in the other direction. That is, one of them toward your head and one away from your head. Always move slowly and methodically while performing these leg variations in *The Shoulder Stand* and count your seconds in each stretch in the same methodical manner that you have learned.

It is very important to keep the back of your head against the floor at all times while coming down out of *The Shoulder Stand*. If you allow your head to leave the floor, you are very liable to roll quickly forward like a ball into a semi-sitting position. This will ruin the slow motion and detract from much of the benefits of the posture. Also, sitting up quickly is not good after having been inverted as in *The Shoulder Stand*. You may arch your head as far back as you have to in order to keep it in contact with the floor while coming out of the posture. Head contact will prevent you from tumbling forward out of control and it will enable you to come out of *The Shoulder Stand* in a beautiful slow motion manner.

If you do not wish to count the time to yourself in the way in which you have been instructed while you are in the posture, you may keep a clock or a watch nearby located in such a manner that you can see it at any time.

# CHAPTER TWENTY-THREE

# Breathing for Beauty
and Health

## About Pranayama

The original texts in Yoga were written thousands of years ago in Sanskrit, the ancient language of India. Pranayama is a very ancient Sanskrit word which means "control of the life-force." The word *yama* means control. The word *Prana* is translated as "life-force."

Pranayama is the Yogic science of breathing that has come down to us unchanged from time immemorial. It consists of a number of specific breathing exercises which have a profound and marvelous effect upon the body, the emotions and the mind.

## The Yoga Concept of Prana or Life-Force

For thousands of years the Yogis and the great scholars, philosophers and thinkers of the East have taught that there is a primal force which permeates the universe. They called this creative force *Prana*. It is the sustainer of all life—plant, animal, and human. When Prana functions in a living creature, that creature is alive. When the Prana or life-force leaves a living thing, that being is dead. On the everyday level, the idea of Prana maintains that:

1. The more Prana a person has, the more fully alive he will be.

2. The more Prana of which a human being can avail himself, the healthier he or she will be.

3. The more Prana people are able to receive, to store within themselves and to use, the more facility they will have toward the attainment of the true goal of human life or the state we refer to in the West as peace of mind.

4. The greatest abundance of Prana available to human beings exists in the atmosphere of the earth.

5. Any human being is able to increase his intake of Prana depending only on his knowledge of how it is done and on his interest and effort.

6. Prana can be stored in the human body. Under average circumstances a person tends to take in about as much Prana as is immediately needed. Actually when a person takes into his body more Prana or life-force than he needs at that particular moment, it is stored in the body for future use. The main place in which it is stored is the region known as the solar plexis, a great nerve center approximately behind the navel in the abdominal region. The solar plexis has sometimes been referred to as the third brain or the brain of the body.

7. Prana is the healer of sickness and is the primary key to health.

8. Prana is available through correct breathing.

9. Prana is more available if correct breathing is combined with right living habits and right use of the mind.

10. Correct eating habits help accumulate Prana because some foods contain more Prana than others, such as fresh organically grown fruits and vegetables, nuts and dried fruits. Some foods are deficient in Prana, including foods that have been tampered with by man, such as canned, frozen, and refined foods, and food products adulterated with chemical preservatives.

## The Effects of Correct Breathing Upon the Body, Emotions and Mind

A change in a person's breathing habits has the ability to change the individual's entire life. Altering one's way of breathing from modern man's shallow hurried little gasps to the deep, full, complete breathing that is normal for a human being, has the ability to improve the total bodily health, improve emotional or mental health, vastly improve the appearance, and promote genuine peace of mind.

Physically, correct breathing purifies the blood, bringing new vigor and life to the entire body. It also results in an improved complexion and strong calm nerves. In addition, we must not overlook the claim made for Yogic breathing that has to do with longevity. It was the Yogis who, centuries ago, observed that those animals in nature which breathe in the shallowest, quickest manner were the most nervous of all creatures and had the shortest life spans as exemplified by the mouse and the rabbit. They observed at the same time that those creatures who breathed long, slow and calm breaths enjoyed the longest lives in the animal kingdom. These included the elephant, the parrot, and the turtle. Yogis themselves are known for their phenomenal life spans and the physical health they enjoy throughout them.

Correct breathing is virtually a necessity if one wishes to have a balanced and truly tranquil emotional makeup. Yogic breathing is the natural healthful way to control the emotions. We all know of the effects of the old "take ten deep breaths" method. That, mind you, is ten simple and nearly always incorrectly performed deep breaths. You will be amazed at the degree of control over your emotions that can be attained by the application of the Yoga breathing exercises. These techniques also have a very strong influence upon bringing about a general positive attitude.

Correct breathing plays an all-important part in the attainment of mind control. The faster and more shallowly you breathe, the more agitated your mind becomes and the more susceptible your emotions are to becoming upset and unbalanced. The slower, deeper and more serenely you breathe, the more your mind will tend to become stable, quieted and tranquil. Correct breathing is the first key to serenity and peace of mind.

## Exercise 29: THE CLEANSING BREATH

STRENGTHENS THE LUNG TISSUE. RIDS THE LUNGS OF HARMFUL IMPURITIES. CLEARS THE MIND. IS AN EXCELLENT AWAKENER IN THE MORNING. RELIEVES COLDS AND CONGESTED NASAL PASSAGES.

### How to practice this exercise

1. Sit erectly in whichever cross-legged position is most comfortable for you.

2. Inhale approximately a third of a lungful of air. Remember to breathe through your nose at all times in Yoga unless instructed otherwise. When performing this partial inhalation, make sure that you expand your abdomen outward as far as you can (Fig. 125).

3. With one sudden vigorous movement pull your abdomen in as swiftly as you can while at the same time you vigorously expel all the air in your lungs through your nostrils. This is a strong movement. Your breath should gush out of your nostrils with considerable noise. The movement should take approximately half a second. The correct performance of the quick exhalation is best described by saying that you should pull

your abdomen in and expel the air out of your nose as if you are being punched in the stomach, the wind being knocked suddenly out of you and escaping forcefully through your nose (Fig. 126).

4. In a more relaxed manner allow your abdomen to expand outwardly again so that the air is sucked quickly back into your lungs through your nostrils. This inhalation should also take approximately half a second (Fig. 125).

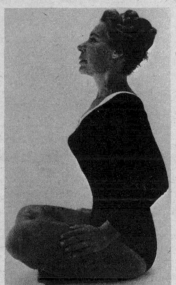

*Figure 125*

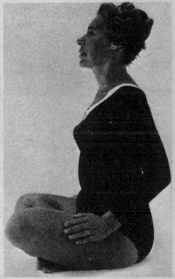

*Figure 126*

5. Repeat the swift vigorous exhalation of Step 3 again. Your abdomen is pulled in forcefully and all the air is expelled from your lungs through your nostrils with a hissing sound.

6. Now repeat the same inhalation procedure as in Step 4. Each separate *Cleansing Breath* consists of one forceful exhalation and one relaxed but equally quick inhalation. Every such *Cleansing Breath* should be performed in approximately one to two seconds.

### Benefits to you

1. *The Cleansing Breath* literally rubs impurities loose from the lung tissue.

2. It relieves colds and numerous symptoms of other common respiratory ailments.

3. Congested nasal passages and sinuses are relieved.

4. The abdomen is developed, making your abdominal wall strong and firm.

5. The diaphragm is strengthened and developed.

6. It strengthens the lungs and strengthens as well as purifies the lung tissue itself.

7. It is a splendid technique for clearing the mind when the mind has become fatigued during the day.

8. It is a superlative "eye opener" for when you wake up in the morning. Nothing can so clear and awaken the mind as a brief round of *Cleansing Breaths* as soon as you sit up in bed in the morning.

### Practice schedule

Ten of these *Cleansing Breaths* (performed in succession one after the other, each *Cleansing Breath* taking approximately 2 seconds to do) equals *one round* of *Cleansing Breaths*.

After each round of 10 *Cleansing Breaths*, take 1 *Complete Breath*.

During the first week you should do 2 rounds of *Cleansing Breaths*. Each round is always followed by 1 *Complete Breath*.

Add 1 round of *Cleansing Breaths* each week until you are doing 6 rounds of *Cleansing Breaths* with each round followed by a *Complete Breath*.

NOTE: An excellent procedure which I recommend is that you perform your *Cleansing Breath* as your first exercise at each Yoga practice session due to its excellent properties of clearing the mind.

### Special hints

There are many impurities in our lungs unless we happen to have lived our entire lives far out in the country. Every hour of every day most of the people in the United States and in other modern industrial countries breathe lungful after lungful of air that is laden with harmful impurities. These range from automobile and bus fumes to the smoke from industrial plants and factories to the awful phenomenon of smog that permeates every cubic inch of air over most of our larger cities. Add to this the frightful intake of poisonous impurities if you happen to be addicted to the cigarette smoking habit. (At the present time the people in New York City, for example, breathe in impurities that are equivalent to smoking two packs of cigarettes a day.) Even if you have lived all your life on the farm, in the country or in some seashore or mountainous locale far from the typical city air pollution, and even if you have not become addicted to cigarettes, certain impurities lodge upon the lung tissue in the form of excessive phlegm and mucus. This is due to improper diet such as the intake of excessively mucus forming foods. All of the impurities which enter and remain in the lungs come to adhere to the sticky tissue there. I have seen an autopsy made of a non-smoker's lung—the lung was white and pure. I have seen the lung itself of a chronic habitual smoker—the lung was hard and dark brown, literally cigar colored.

I am painting a bleak picture in order to drive home the urgent necessity for practicing the breathing techniques that you are taught here so that you can combat the truly major problem of the intake of impurities into our most tender and vital organ. Many people—millions I am sure—further add to the intake of harmful and often poisonous impurities of the lungs by the bad breathing habit known as mouth breathing.

The mouth breathing habit is very harmful. Many people breathe through their mouths inadvertently while sleeping. Others also inadvertently do so during their waking day. The air that is drawn into your lungs through your mouth is unfiltered air. The nasal passages are composed of mucus membranes with many small hairs. This structure is designated by nature to filter the air you breathe so that a percentage of impurities does not go directly to your bronchial tubes and lungs.

The impurities you breathe are harmful and destructive to the lungs. They drain your vitality and make you more susceptible to chronic fatigue. They can indeed be considered as indirect contributory factors toward mental depression.

All the Yoga breathing techniques are of great aid in helping you overcome the cigarette habit. I have had students in my classes tell me that after six months of applying themselves sincerely to the breathing techniques they developed an aversion to cigarettes and were thus able to break the habit.

I maintain that if applied correctly, the Yoga breathing exercises can so purify the lungs that cigarette smoke becomes repugnant to the individual. The lungs themselves rebel against the intake of cigarette smoke and its accompanying poisons such as nicotine and coal tar. Nothing can so purify and strengthen the lungs, and offset all these negative factors in our civilization of which we have just spoken, than the diligent practice of *The Cleansing Breath* in combination with *The Complete Breath* which you are now going to learn.

This combination of-breathing exercises (10 *Cleansing Breaths* followed by one *Complete Breath*) can and should be practiced a number of times during the day. Fortunately, it is a procedure that can be performed at nearly any time. When no one is watching you, you can do it at work or while driving your car, while waiting, and even unnoticed while walking along the street. You can perform it in your home many times. I cannot urge you too strongly to do so. Simply remember whenever you do it during the day to adhere to the practice schedule that you are using in your regular formal daily workout. For example, if you are performing four rounds of *Cleansing Breaths,* each one followed by a *Complete Breath,* as you would be in the third week of practice, then do only that many at each time when you decide to engage in this healthful breathing practice.

## Exercise 30: THE COMPLETE BREATH

DEVELOPS THE CHEST, DIAPHRAGM AND LUNGS.
PURIFIES THE BLOOD THROUGH INCREASED OXY-
GEN INTAKE. INCREASES RESISTANCE TO COLDS.

### *How to practice this exercise*

1. Sit in a cross-legged position on your mat. Breathe normally. Now pull your abdomen in and at the same time exhale through your nose until your lungs are empty. This movement is in preparation for *The Complete Breath.*

2. Begin *The Complete Breath* by inhaling slowly, smoothly and quietly through your nose. At the same time that you inhale, push your abdomen out as far as you possibly can. Push your abdomen out as little children do when they attempt to "make a big belly." Abdominal expansion is of uppermost importance. By pushing your abdomen outward, you cause your diaphragm to stretch downward. The diaphragm is a sheet of muscles just underneath the lungs. When the diaphragm moves downward, it gives the bottom portion of the lungs room to expand. Thus, by the outward movement of your abdomen, the air you inhale is able to go directly to the bottom portion of the lungs so that it can begin filling the lungs completely from the bottom.

This part of your inhalation in which you expand your abdomen should take 5 seconds (Fig. 125).

3. Still inhaling through your nose in a smooth continuous manner,

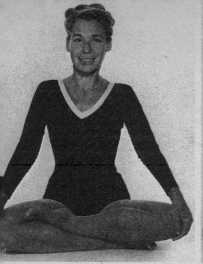
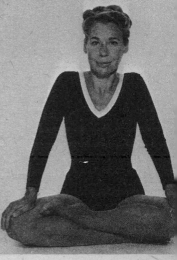

*Figure 127*

*Figure 128*

pull your abdomen slowly in while at the same time you expand your chest. Expand your chest by pushing forward with your breastbone and spreading your ribs. This part of your inhalation should take you another 5 seconds (Fig. 127).

It should take you 10 seconds in all to accomplish one complete inhalation of breath.

4. Raise your shoulders slightly and hold the breath you have taken for 5 seconds (Fig. 128).

5. To exhale, simply begin exhaling through your nose relaxing your shoulders and chest as you do so. Keep your abdomen pulled in firmly throughout the entire holding and exhalation of your breath.

It should take you 10 seconds to exhale.

6. When your breath has been exhaled entirely from your body, your abdomen will be pulled in firmly and you are ready to repeat the entire *Complete Breath* once more.

7. Summary of *The Complete Breath:* Inhale a smooth, slow, quiet breath for 10 seconds. During the first 5 seconds of your inhalation, expand your abdomen slowly outward as far as it can go. During the next 5 seconds of your inhalation, pull your abdomen slowly in and expand your chest as much as you are able. Hold your breath for 5 seconds. Exhale for 10 seconds with your abdomen held firmly in. The only time your abdomen expands outward in *The Complete Breath* is during the first half of your inhalation.

### Benefits to you

1. The effects of *The Complete Breath* upon the body are such that the person who practices the exercise, especially as part of a full Yoga exercise schedule, will soon develop a noticeable glow of renewed health and radiant beauty.

2. *The Complete Breath* develops and expands the entire chest in supple lines.

3. It enriches and purifies the blood because of the increased intake of oxygen into the lungs. This is of incalculable benefit to your health and beauty.

4. *The Complete Breath* increases resistance to colds and other common respiratory conditions.

5. The nervous system is strengthened and calmed.

6. It strengthens and develops the diaphragm for a flat "tummy."

7. Increased clarity and alertness of mind are induced.

8. It increases the intake of Prana or life-force into all your organs which brings all the wonderful effects of which we have spoken.

### Practice schedule

Perform *The Complete Breath* after every round (10 breaths) of *The Cleansing Breath*.

It is a very good practice to conclude your exercise period with at least 3 complete breaths.

*The Complete Breath* was also meant to be practiced at any time throughout the day or evening. The more you do it the more of its effects you will receive and the better off you will be. If you practice *The Complete Breath* during the day whenever you feel the need for it, you can, according to the circumstances, eliminate the holding of the breath. In this way it is a splendid exercise to perform while driving your car and especially while walking. I strongly urge you to practice *The Complete Breath* whenever you are walking. At that time you should coordinate the count with the steps that you take. For example, you would inhale for 10 steps, hold your breath for 5, and exhale for 10. The combination of walking plus *The Complete Breath* is one of the most superlatively healthful activities that you can possibly engage in.

Here is a very important point to remember. The counting is designated to make you adhere to a certain ratio—the 10:5:10 (or 2:1:2) ratio. If, as you progress in your practice of Yoga, you feel the inclination to lengthen the inhalation, holding and exhalation of *The Complete Breath*, do so by simply slowing down your count. In other words, only in the beginning will your count of 10 have to adhere to that number of seconds. Later on your count of 10 may actually be 20 or more seconds. It is a matter of holding your original ratio of inhalation to retention to exhalation.

When you are accustomed to the exercise and wish to increase your breath retention, you may increase the ratio to 10:10:10. That is, inhale for the count of 10, hold your breath for the count of 10, and exhale for the count of 10. I recommend that you perform the original 10:5:10 count for at least one month before you increase the time of breath retention.

### Special hints

A school teacher who took our course in Hatha Yoga told us that she had taught *The Complete Breath* to her fourth grade class. She said that she had originally taught it to them as a part of their general education so that they should know what correct breathing is and how to do it. As she went on, however, she found that she would have them perform *The Complete Breath* during the times of the school day when they became restless, nervous or agitated. She informed us that she has never in all her teaching experience found anything that could so quickly, so efficiently and so pleasantly calm down an entire class of thirty nine-year-old children.

The Yoga breathing exercises are of prime importance in counteracting the fumes and impurities which we breathe in our age of fallout. It is also indispensable in counteracting the nearly universal bad habit of high or shallow breathing. Most people breathe with the upper third or quarter of their lungs, making no use whatever of all the rest of their lungs. The effects of the high fast breathing habit are devastating. It results in a devitalization of the body, chronic fatigue, lack of energy and susceptibility to mental depression.

*The Complete Breath* is man's natural way of breathing. By re-educating your body to breathe in this manner (and it is a simple delightful process to do so) you are relearning the original instinctive way of breathing of the human species before our breathing habits were impaired by tension and other conditions.

## What Happens to the Abdomen

I have stressed in the instructions the reason for expanding the abdomen. The principle behind expanding the abdomen (to lower the diaphragm and thus to give the lower portion of the lung room to expand) is exemplified in the image of filling a paper bag. If the bottom of a paper bag is crumpled or closed, whatever enters the bag will not fill the bag up from the bottom but will begin filling it from wherever the bag is open and free. When you lower the diaphragm and thus allow the bottom of the lungs to expand, it is like opening the bag completely before attempting to fill it. The air that you breathe in this manner travels to the bottom of the lungs and fills them completely.

## Some Special Points on the Complete Breath

I would like to list a few points regarding *The Complete Breath* which you should bear in mind.

1. All breathing is done through the nose.

2. The body movements, mainly of the abdomen and chest, should be done smoothly and rhythmically and they should flow into each other as if it is all one movement.

3. Your breath itself should be one continuous inhalation: smooth, even and unwavering.

4. In *The Complete Breath* you should inhale and exhale silently so that you cannot hear your breath going in and out of your body. This aids in slowing down your breathing and is quieting and soothing for the mind.

5. At the end of *The Complete Breath* when you have exhaled all the air from your lungs, you should pull your abdomen in and up tightly in order to squeeze the last of the carbon dioxide, old air and impurities from them.

6. Close your eyes while performing *The Complete Breath* and think of nothing but the movements of your body and of your breath moving in and out of your body. This in itself is excellent preparatory practice for a mental technique which you will later learn for the attaining of peace of mind.

You should become accustomed to think of breathing as a form of nourishment just as you think of eating or drinking as a form of nourishment. You can go without eating for a month or more and you will probably receive nothing but good benefits from such abstention. The body can survive without water for nearly a week. However, if you stop taking air into your body you will perish within minutes. Surely then, we can see that air and all that it carries, oxygen and Prana, is the primary form of human nourishment. We are simply not accustomed to thinking of it in that way. Be aware that with every breath you are feeding yourself with life's most vital sustenance. Do not allow yourself to starve for this primary food of life due to incomplete breathing.

# CHAPTER TWENTY-FOUR

# A Yoga Technique
# for Calming the Nerves
# and Improving Sleep

## Modern Civilization's Problem of Nervousness

The problem of nerves that exists in our modern civilization certainly warrants the concern given to it by both medical authorities and by the average man. The condition called "nerves" is really a major malady in our time and especially in the United States. It may exist to such an extent in an individual as to result, in time, in heart attacks. Mostly, however, it is a chronic condition that has become part of the lives of tens of millions of people.

The symptoms include general irritability, jumpiness, and an inability to be calm and relaxed. While the word "nerves" is often used to cover up a lack of knowledge of exactly what may be wrong with a person, there is no doubt whatsoever that the condition exists on an individual basis and more and more as a national illness.

There is a kind of living for the future which goes beyond the normal "planning toward a goal" that is a wholesome part of everyday life. Many persons have fallen so far into the quagmire of their desires and ambitions that they are no longer able to enjoy the present moment of living at all. This can develop to the degree of being a psychological aberration. In many instances obsessive preoccupation with the future becomes no more than a retreat from the fact of being incapable of living now. In any case, man was meant to live fully now, in the eternal present, and when he goes too far on the path of performing his actions for a future attainment, he runs a serious risk of nervous or psychological breakdown.

If we can learn to live in closer contact with nature, develop a serenity that can cope with all kinds of personalities, devote more time to filling our personal life and immediate environment with beauty, and engage in really fulfilling recreational activities, the world would change for us from a tense harried one to one in which we lived in harmony with ourselves, other people and our environment. *Yoga was conceived to produce this change,* a change within you from nervousness to calm, from strife to harmony, from tension to serenity.

## About Sleep

For many people the problem of nerves makes itself felt in regard to their sleep. We can scarcely calculate the number of people in our country who have difficulty falling asleep, who do not get any rest out of their sleep or who are victims of actual insomnia. There are certain facts regarding sleep which are necessary to know before the problem can be corrected.

## Sleep Cycles Vary

The first thing to realize is that different people have different sleep cycles. Some people are natural early-to-bed-and-early-to-rise individuals. They can only really thrive if they are able to maintain this type of sleep schedule. These persons are very fortunate because our culture is generally geared to their cycle. Other people are the exact opposite. They are natural night workers. They are people whose cycle is to sleep very late in the day, if not most of the day, and to be up most or all of the night. I know many persons of this nature, some of whom are fortunate enough to be in an occupation which is in harmony with their sleep cycle. There are other persons whose natural sleep cycle is to go to bed late, to get up early, to thrive quite well but to need a nap in the afternoon. These people are under a continual physical and psychological strain if they have to live according to the nine to five work schedule which typifies so great a part of our society. There are other persons whose natural sleep cycle is such that no matter what time they go to sleep, whether it be early in the evening or very late at night, they have to sleep until, let us say, nine-thirty in the morning. If they get up before that particular time their nerves are on edge, their day is marred and their efficiency in their occupation is lowered. These are morning sleepers whose soundest rest takes place from dawn through mid-morning.

Due to the way society is organized and the obligation of working in accord with its pattern, an enormous number of people are not able to sleep according to their natural sleep cycle. What these people must do then is to make certain that the *quality* of their sleep is of the highest possible level so that at least, when they do sleep, they get the most out of it. Sleeping correctly, deeply and in the most relaxed physical, emotional and mental way possible is sufficient to overcome a considerable portion of the problem of nerves.

## Why People Sleep Imperfectly

Most people sleep imperfectly. For one thing they go to sleep physically tense. They carry their day and all its problems with them into sleep with all its physical, nervous, emotional and mental jangling. Most people cannot stop their minds from revolving around and around from the moment they lay down to the moment that they mercifully fall asleep. Your body remains tense throughout the night. Your physical organism is reacting to thoughts that relate to the day's problems. You wonder why you wake up tired and feeling miserable in the morning, often as exhausted as when you lay your head down upon your pillow to sleep. Obviously such sleep did you little good.

In just describing the sleep problem, I have described part of the problem of insomnia. I will only add that the insomniac spends many of his hours of torture in thinking and worrying about the fact that he is not able to sleep. In a rather ironical way this makes insomnia the cause of insomnia. Intense preoccupation combined with other thoughts that are nagging repetitiously through the mind constitute a vicious cycle which keeps the insomniac awake.

I have often advised persons who complain of insomnia to go along with it; that is, to ride along with the sleeplessness, to stop worrying or caring about whether they sleep or not and to simply let the mind wander on while they lie there watching it as if they were watching a movie. A great many of these people have returned to inform me that their ceasing to care about whether they were able to sleep or not relieved their anxiety and their condition to a very great degree, and they fell asleep much sooner than usual.

This technique, however, is only a minor aid to relieving the problem of insomnia. It requires the *Alternate Nostril Breathing* exercise of Yoga to really solve the problem.

## Yoga and Tranquility

The quantity of tranquilizers taken every year in the United States is staggering to conceive in terms of danger to health and in terms of countless millions of dollars spent. What does a person gain from a tranquilizer pill? He obtains a brief interval of partial pacification. This tranquility is of a superficial nature and has no lasting positive effect. It has, rather, cumulative negative effects upon body, mind and character and in no way teaches or enables the user to attain peace of mind or tranquility in the future. Once knowing the *Alternate Nostril Breathing* technique—especially when practiced in conjunction with a daily schedule of Yoga stretching exercises—a person need never take a tranquilizer again.

To be free from nervousness two things are necessary. First, you must be able to put your body in a state of genuine relaxation, the state which is reached by the practice of the Yoga stretching techniques. The second requirement is that you must sleep normally.

To sleep correctly you must go to sleep already relaxed to a very great extent. Your nerves must already be tranquilized, your emotions must be calmed and stabilized, and your mind must be used correctly and in proper condition before you fall asleep. These are the requirements for deep and therapeutic sleep: the kind of sleep that nourishes the tissue of the nervous system itself, rests the entire body, rests the heart, emotions and mind and which rejuvenates your entire physical—mental organism. Thus we see that the pre-sleep state of mind and body is of the utmost importance.

*The Alternate Nostril Breathing* exercise which you are going to learn now is the most perfect and efficient natural technique known to the human race for wiping clean the tensions, nervousness and anxieties which have come to occupy your mind and body from the pressures and responsibilities of the day.

## Exercise 31: ALTERNATE NOSTRIL BREATHING

CALMS BOTH BODY AND MIND. IS THE KEY TO
EMOTIONAL CONTROL. HELPS OVERCOME NEGA-
TIVE EMOTIONS SUCH AS FEAR, WORRY AND
ANXIETY. STRENGTHENS THE NERVOUS SYSTEM.
IS OF GREAT AID IN OVERCOMING INSOMNIA.
IMPARTS THE FEELING AND AIR OF SERENITY.

### How to practice this exercise

1. Sit erectly in a cross-legged position on your mat. If you can sit comfortably in *The Half Lotus* or in *The Full Lotus,* it is advisable to do so. Otherwise *The Simple Posture* will do quite well.

2. Place your right hand in the position that is indicated in Fig. 129. That is: the tips of your index finger and middle finger are placed against your forehead between your eyebrows; your right thumb rests lightly

against your right nostril without closing that nostril; your ring finger rests lightly against your left nostril also without closing your nostril; your little finger is alongside your ring finger. Exhale as much air as you can through your nostrils emptying your lungs.

3. Press down upon your right nostril with your right thumb. Lift your ring finger from your left nostril and begin to breathe in through your left nostril. Fill your lungs, using the body movement of *The Complete Breath*, by inhaling through your left nostril for the count of 8 (Fig. 130).

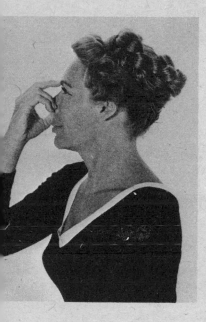

*Figure 129*

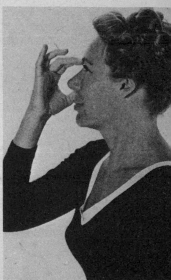

*Figure 130*

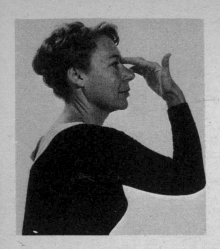

*Figure 131*

4. Press your ring finger down upon your left n stril so that both nostrils are closed. Hold your breath for the count of 4.

5. Raise your right thumb off your right nostril and exhale through your right nostril for the count of 8. Make sure that you exhale all the air from your lungs during this count (Fig. 131).

6. Without changing the position of your hands, immediately breathe in through your right nostril for the count of 8.

7. Press your right thumb down upon your right nostril so that both nostrils are tightly closed. Hold your breath for the count of 4.

8. Lift your ring finger from your left nostril again and exhale through that nostril for the count of 8.

9. The movements you have just performed while breathing 2 *Complete Breaths* constitute "one round" of *Alternate Nostril Breathing*.

At this point you will repeat the *Alternate Nostril Breathing* technique for as many rounds as are prescribed under the Practice Schedule.

### Benefits to you

1. *Alternate Nostril Breathing* calms the nerves. This is not a superficial effect, but a very profound tranquilization, and without tranquilizer pills.

2. It is of inestimable aid in combating and overcoming insomnia.

3. It produces an immediate calming effect upon the body, providing a great relief from agitation and physical irritability.

4. The nervous system is strengthend to cope with any situation.

5. It is the key to emotional control and is of enormous practical value in calming and controlling upset emotions.

6. It is of great aid in overcoming negative emotions such as grief, anger, fear and worry that scar your beauty.

7. It has the ability to develop the characteristic of even-temperedness, serenity at its best.

8. It quiets the mind, conserves its power.

9. It develops the habit and the trait of serenity in the midst of even the most chaotic situations.

10. *Alternate Nostril Breathing* brings an increased amount of Prana or life-force into the body which affects its ability to strengthen the nervous system.

11. It is a valuable aid in overcoming many nervous conditions.

12. When you have a headache, by all means practice *Alternate Nostril Breathing*. I am continually being told by students in the most enthusiastic terms of the remarkably soothing effects of this exercise upon headaches.

### Practice schedule

During the first week of practice you should adhere to the 8:4:8 ratio. That is, inhale for the count of 8, hold for the count of 4, exhale for the count of 8.

After this, for a period of 1 month, you should hold to an 8:8:8 ratio. That is the count that you should practice if you are inclined to need or simply desire *Alternate Nostril Breathing* while in the midst of the activities of the world such as while waiting or while driving a car, if you can perform it at these times unobserved by other people.

In any case it is essential for your health, emotional tranquility, mental quietude and appearance to practice formally at home in a quiet, private place every day.

In your regular Yoga exercise period at home you should do 7 rounds of *Alternate Nostril Breathing*.

## Advanced Techniques

The 8:8:8 ratio is sufficient for the purposes that have been described. If, however, you wish to advance, you may do so in the following manner. After at least 1 month of practicing at an 8:8:8 count, you may change the count to 8:8:16. That is, inhale for the count of 8, retain your breath for the count of 8, and exhale for the count of 16. This is as far as you should go by yourself. If you wish to advance even further, you should seek the personal instruction of a qualified Yoga teacher.

By all means, however, practice this exercise. Attempt to do a full

7 rounds when you have retired for the night. When the lights are out and you are lying comfortably in bed upon your back, then is the time to wipe away the nervous, emotional and the mental tensions of the day so that you can sleep deeply and correctly. After a while the effect is so long lasting that you begin to wake up in the morning feeling truly rested, re-energized and at the same time in a serene and positive state of mind.

### Special hints

There is a story that comes down to us from centuries ago in India. It is about a nobleman who fell into disfavor with the king and was imprisoned in a high stone tower. The only opening in his cell was a small window but it was of no avail to the prisoner because of the long drop to the ground. One night his wife came to the bottom of the tower and called up to him, "Is there anything I can do?"

"Yes," he answered. "Come back tomorrow night and bring with you a drop of honey, a beetle, a long spool of fine thread, a long spool of strong cord, and a long coil of rope." Puzzled she went and did as he told her. The next night she appeared at the base of the tower. "Did you bring everything?" he asked. "Yes, husband," she said. "Very well," he told her. "Tie the end of the thread around the middle of the beetle." She did so. "Now put the drop of honey on the end of the beetle's horns." "It is done." "Good," he replied. "Now place the beetle on the wall and point him upward." She did so and immediately the beetle began to walk up following the scent of the honey that was on his own horns. The beetle walked up the length of the tower and eventually the prisoner was able to grasp it. When he did so he took hold of the thread. "Now," he said to his wife, "Tie the cord on the end of the thread." When she did this he pulled the thread up until he could grasp hold of the cord. "Now," he said, "Tie the rope to the end of the cord." She did so. He pulled the rope up, tied one end of it in his cell, climbed down it and thus escaped.

One of the foremost meanings given to the tale is that the thread represents the breath and that by means of a little thread one can, with wisdom, bring about the rope from which to escape imprisonment. The imprisonment is none other than one's imprisonment in a multitude of personal problems that ultimately add up to what we can call lack of peace of mind.

## The Body-Mind Entity

The body and mind, as we are well aware, are not two separate entities. It is now realized that body and mind are two parts or aspects of one complete organism. They are simply composed of different form and substance. What happens to the mind happens to the body and what happens to the body happens to the mind. They affect and influence each other in a very direct manner.

Some doctors maintain that the physical symptoms of over seventy percent of all of their patients are of mental origin. The most obvious standard case is that of ulcers. Ulcers are to the greater extent the direct result of a nervous condition which is brought about by worry and emotional strain. There is no micro-organism causing that hole to be eaten in the stomach lining.

What we have overlooked, however, is that the reverse is also true. The body has a direct and powerful effect upon the mind as is especially apparent when the body is in pain. It is the mind that suffers and is unable to function normally. In normal conditions the body is continually affecting the mind. When the body is run down and in a weak, fatigued, nervous, tense, debilitated condition, the mind will be upset, agitated and susceptible to depression, anxiety, fear and worry. When a person conversely subjects their body to a healthful regime of relaxing and invigorating exercises, the first effects upon the mind are delight, clarity, cheer and increased efficiency.

## Old Ideas of Breath Control Over Emotions

We are all aware of the common practice of taking "ten deep breaths" when upset emotionally, and we all know it works. If you have to appear on stage, if you have to go to see the boss, if you receive bad news, or if you have just had an argument, taking ten deep breaths will certainly contribute to soothing your upset nerves and emotions. Thus, we see, that the breath has a direct control over the nervous system and the emotions.

## Scientific Breath Control Over Emotions

If ten commonplace deep breaths, performed incorrectly, without control, proper training or knowledge and without the breaths even being complete, can begin to assuage a force as powerful as overwrought emotions, can you conceive of the result in regard to balancing the emotions that such a scientific and perfect technique as *Alternate Nostril Breathing* can have.

No natural movement known to man has the incredibly powerful, direct and immediate effect upon soothing and tranquilizing the nerves and emotional states as *Alternate Nostril Breathing*. The very technique itself is designed to balance certain positive and negative currents that flow through the human body. The profundity of this breathing technique alone can be the material for an entire separate study by anyone who wishes to go deeper into the subject of Yoga.

Here are certain points to always remember when performing the *Alternate Nostril Breathing* exercise.

Keep your posture erect when you are sitting to perform this technique.

Do not allow the air to gush out when you exhale if you can possibly help it. The more perfectly you control your exhalation and the closer you adhere to the rhythmical pattern of your count the better the result will be.

Besides practicing *Alternate Nostril Breathing* as part of your regular daily Yoga workout, you should do it whenever you are upset or whenever you are going to go into a situation which you feel will make you nervous.

Always remember to use *The Complete Breath* throughout the *Alternate Nostril Breathing*.

When practicing the breath retention, it is a good practice as soon as you begin holding your breath to lower your head so that your chin rests upon the jugular notch just above your sternum or breast bone. When your breath retention is over, raise your head, slowly of course, in order to begin your exhalation.

# CHAPTER TWENTY-FIVE

# The Problem of
# Regularity Solved

## The Causes of Irregularity

Irregularity is at least a chronic nuisance and inconvenience to an individual, and it is just as often a major health problem. It is so widespread a condition that it is definitely a health problem of a national scale. Witness the millions of dollars spent every year on patent laxatives. Besides the immediate inconvenience to the victim, the main negative aspect of it is the danger to a person's health that can come from the long term self-poisoning which comes from improper regularity.

There are two main general causes of irregularity. One has to do with our eating habits. The other involves lack of proper use of our body.

In regard to eating there is no doubt that the situation of devitalized foods which exists in our country today is a major cause of irregularity. Many people haven't eaten a piece of tree, vine or farm ripened fruit or vegetable in years. So much of our food is canned, frozen or otherwise tampered with that an alarming percentage of nutritional value is gone. All too often persons suffering from irregularity are eating exactly the wrong foods for their condition. For example, a high carbohydrate diet with much bread and potatoes is the worst thing one can eat in cases of irregularity. There is no doubt that the irregularity problem can be cured or at least alleviated by correct eating. Fruit juices, fresh fruits and vegetables and staying away from constipating foods such as starches can work wonders.

The lack of normal vigorous physical activity in the lives of most modern people also causes irregularity. Millions of persons with sedentary or inactive jobs are primary victims. Exercise, especially of a scientific nature such as Yoga, activates the internal organs so they function normally.

For the greater part irregularity is the result of impaired peristaltic action, known in popular terms as "sluggish colon." Peristaltic action is a wavelike motion which is continually taking place throughout the entire length of our alimentary canal. The alimentary canal is that tube which begins at the throat and consists of the esophagus, stomach, the small intestines and the colon. Though this tube takes different shapes along its path and though its sections perform vastly different functions, it is nonetheless one continuous tube. Along it there continually proceeds a wavelike motion which propels food substances from mouth to colon. The wave-like motion is what is responsible for our ability to swallow food, for example, while we are upside down, propelling the food against the very force of gravity. It is absolutely essential that the peristaltic action be normally healthful and vigorous throughout the colon or large intestine. Due to devitalized foods, eating of wrong food combinations and improper use of the body such as lack of regular exercise, movement becomes sluggish in the large intestine. Thus, because movement is improper, we have the uncomfortable, unhealthy and dangerous condition known as irregularity.

## The Dangers of Laxatives

Since this condition is so widespread nationally, we find ourselves bombarded continually with advertisements for laxatives. Most people have come to think of laxatives as the only solution. What is worse, laxatives have come to be part of the way of life of millions of people and are accepted as simply another necessity.

Laxatives, however, are not the simple solution to the problem as they would seem on the surface. Most laxatives are nothing more than an unnatural and even a somewhat poisonous substance. In the body's desperate attempt to eliminate this negative and undesirable substance it eliminates the contents of the colon indiscriminately. Other laxatives, while not as overtly toxic, are excessively harsh and temporarily stimulate the colon to do its work. No laxative can ever really cure the problem of irregularity. They can only offer temporary relief of an artificial, unnatural nature. The worst thing that they do, however, is to weaken the ability of the colon to function on its own accord. The more we take them the more the colon comes to depend upon that external means. In time the colon grows weaker and weaker because of the laxative and eventually can scarcely function at all without it. The individual is then one of the innumerable victims of laxative addiction. They dare not stop taking the laxative for it is the only thing that can aid them to eliminate. This is the gravest danger of laxatives.

## The Yoga Solution to Irregularity

Altering the diet is one solution but a person is usually not able to alter it sufficiently to completely cure the problem. Another solution is a daily Yoga exercise regime which includes the incredible exercise, *The Abdominal Contraction*. This, in my opinion, is the most perfect solution to the problem of irregularity.

*The Abdominal Contraction* is a bodily movement whose specific function is to stimulate sluggish peristaltic action back to its normal, dependable, regular activity. The results I have seen have been nothing less than astonishing.

### Exercise 32: THE ABDOMINAL CONTRACTION

RESTORES PROPER PERISTALTIC ACTION IN THE COLON. MASSAGES AND STIMULATES VITAL IN-TERNAL GLANDS AND ORGANS.

#### How to practice this exercise

1. Stand with your heels at about shoulder width apart and with your feet at a slight outward angle. Bend your legs at the knees until you are in approximately a one-quarter squat. Place your palms on your thighs, about halfway between your knees and your groin, with your fingers pointing toward the insides of your thighs. Now, without moving your body from the hips down, allow as much of your weight as you can to be supported by your arms. You are supporting the weight of your upper body upon your thighs. This should give you a slightly relaxed or hanging feeling in your abdomen. Your shoulders will be a little higher than usual. You are now in the basic position for *The Abdominal Contraction*. See Fig. 132.

2. Exhale *all* the air out of your lungs through your mouth. Make a whistling sound through your pursed lips as you exhale. Hold your breath *out* of your lungs throughout the following movements.

3. With the air being held *out* of your lungs, pull in and upward with your abdomen. Remember not to allow yourself to inhale any air whatsoever while performing these movements.

4. By pulling up in this manner you will create the great hollow indentation in your abdominal region that is shown in Fig. 133. (If you

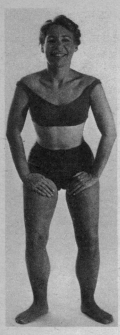

Figure 132

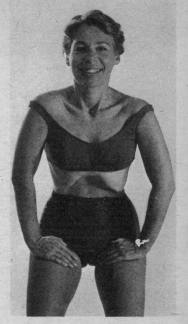

Figure 133

are overweight around your abdomen or waist you may not see the indentation occurring right away.) Hold the position for the count of 1.

5. After holding the inward and upward pull for the count of 1, pop your abdomen back out with a vigorous though not violent movement.

6. After popping your abdomen back out in a brisk manner, suck it vigorously back in and up again. Repeat the exact same in and out movement four more times so that you will have performed *The Abdominal Contraction* 5 times on one breath exhalation. That is: position; exhalation; in-out, in-out, in-out, in-out, in-out. This is called 1 set of 5 *Abdominal Contractions*.

7. Stand up erectly and inhale. Catch your breath until you are breathing normally once again. Your body will quickly adapt itself to this form of breathing.

8. Return to your starting position and in the same manner do another set of 5 *Abdominal Contractions* according to the practice schedule that will be given.

9. Let me summarize. Position, exhalation, do 5 *Abdominal Contractions* without inhaling any air, stand up and catch your breath, repeat the procedure.

### Benefits to you

1. *The Abdominal Contraction* relieves constipation and restores regularity by stimulating and normalizing the peristaltic action of the colon.

2. The abdominal muscles are strengthened and abdominal weight is reduced.

3. It greatly aids in reducing weight around the waist.

4. *The Abdominal Contraction* stimulates and massages the internal organs such as the colon, small intestines, sexual glands, kidneys, liver, gall bladder and pancreas.

5. It helps restore a dropped abdomen to normal condition.

### Practice schedule

Perform *The Abdominal Contraction* in an even rhythmical manner. Pull in and up for the count of 1, pop your abdomen back out for the count of 1.

Your progress should adhere to the following pattern.

First day: 5 sets of 5 contractions.
Second day: 6 sets of 5 contractions.
Third day: 7 sets of 5 contractions.
Fourth day: 8 sets of 5 contractions.
Fifth day: 9 sets of 5 contractions.
Sixth day: 10 sets of 5 contractions.

At this point you will be doing 50 *Abdominal Contractions* which should take you about 2 minutes or less to perform. Imagine the great benefit to your health in these mere 2 minutes. Fifty *Abdominal Contractions* will be sufficient for you if your regularity is normal or reasonably close to normal.

You should do 50 *Abdominal Contractions* at least once a day. The best time is in the morning on an empty stomach, before breakfast. I recommend, however, that you repeat your schedule of *Abdominal Contractions* 3 times a day. You must always practice it on an empty stomach. The best times are before meals. If it is not practical for you to exercise before meals, then make sure that you have not eaten for at least two hours.

If you have a more serious problem with constipation or irregularity and if your physician has verified that it is simply irregularity and not an actual pathological condition, or if you simply wish to go on to a more advanced level in Hatha Yoga, you may feel perfectly confident in increasing your *Abdominal Contractions* according to the following pattern.

Seventh day: 10 sets of 6 contractions.
Eighth day: 10 sets of 7 contractions.
Ninth day: 10 sets of 8 contractions.
Tenth day: 10 sets of 9 contractions.
Eleventh day: 10 sets of 10 contractions.

By advancing to this level it means that it will take you from 2 to 4 minutes to perform your *Abdominal Contractions* at any one time. Again, you should exercise at least once a day before breakfast and then repeat the exercise 3 times a day.

### Special hints

There is no other way outside of Yoga to actually reach into the abdominal region and affect in a positive way the vital organs and glands that are contained there. *The Abdominal Contraction* is a completely natural movement and it is the greatest natural movement known to man for directly working out and promoting the health of the internal organs.

When a person's abdomen becomes flabby and out of condition it tends to sag. When the abdominal wall sags—because the muscles are deteriorated—then all the organs which are normally held in correctly also sag out of place. When the visceral organs sag out of place, their functions become impaired producing a dangerous condition. It is a rule of nature that any part of the body which is not moved or used as nature meant it to be will deteriorate. If you tied your arm down to your side so that you could not use it for months it would begin to atrophy and wither. If you prevented it from being used long enough, you could reach the day where you would never be able to use it again. The same applies to all our body parts. *The Abdominal Contraction* reconditions and firms the abdominal wall and helps bring your vital internal organs back into their proper high position. Its massaging and stimulating effect produces a complete internal and external reconditioning of your abdominal area.

The importance of holding your breath entirely out of your lungs during the exercise is that the diaphragm is raised and a vacuum formed into which the visceral organs are rhythmically pulled. This lifting motion raises the organs and stretches the colon and intestines. It is the pulling or stretching movement that stimulates and restores the normal peristaltic action to the colon.

People with a history of a cardiac condition should consult their physician before practicing this technique because in certain cases of heart condition it is not advisable to hold the breath out. If, however, your heart is normal this exercise can only produce good results.

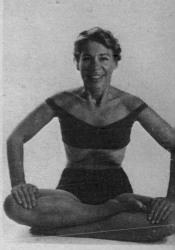

Figure 135

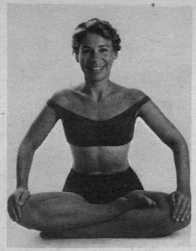

Figure 134

If you are overweight in your waist or your abdomen, keep on practicing the exercise. In time you will note great improvement in that area.

The proper way of performing the contraction comes in time. You will quickly get the "feel" of it. It is a pulling in and at the same time a raising up of the abdominal portion of your body.

Those who wish to attack the problem of constipation and irregularity more seriously may try the following for a few days. Drink a small glass of water with the juice of half a lemon squeezed in it before performing the exercise.

Observe yourself in a mirror as you practice *The Abdominal Contraction*. When you see the great hollow indentation in your abdomen and at the same time a hollow spot appear in the lower notch of your throat, you will know that you are performing it correctly. I recommend that you take a *Complete Breath* when catching your breath after each set.

*The Abdominal Contraction* can be practiced sitting down with the same results. When sitting, simply press in against your knees with your hands to help raise your abdomen correctly. See Fig. 134 and Fig. 135.

193

# CHAPTER TWENTY-SIX

# Increasing Balance,
# Poise and Grace

A charming woman is standing in a public place. She is shapely, has a pretty face and is dressed attractively. She moves toward a chair and sits down. The image of beauty she projected at first sight is shattered like a pane of glass. She moved as clumsily as a typical country bumpkin.

A chic young woman walks across the room at a party. You might as well cancel out all the lovely qualities of her face, form and dress. There is something about her walk that is strangely reminiscent of a longshoreman . . . or is it a nine-year-old tom-boy.

There is no counting how many times I have seen women's beauty marred by deficient grace. It is the life we lead as modern people that detracts from the grace and poise that nature meant us to have. Our lack of normal physical activity results in the diminishing of our sense of balance, and it is this loss of the normal sense of balance that is responsible for the impairment of grace and poise.

Never being called upon to use your sense of balance to its full capacity, it deteriorates. Athletes possess this balance. That is why athletes often have what is called a "cat-like grace." *When a person's poise and grace are lessened, her self-confidence is damaged whether she is conscious of it or not.* A more serious condition than the loss of a certain degree of beauty, it can have far reaching negative effects upon your life.

What you must do is reverse the process of deterioration by restoring the sense of balance to its full natural condition. The result is the regaining of natural poise and grace and consequently the increasing of self-confidence. A feeling of lightness also develops from improved balance and grace revealing itself in every movement of your body and in the air about you.

Certain Yoga exercises are particularly excellent at accomplishing the restoration of balance and all the significant qualities that come with it. *The Arm and Leg Stretch* is most notable among these exercises.

### Exercise 33: THE ARM AND LEG STRETCH

#### *How to practice this exercise*

1. Stand erectly with your hands at your sides, chest high, abdomen in, and your feet together.

2. Slowly raise your right arm into the air until it is above your head but not altogether perpendicular.

3. Place all your weight on your right leg.

4. Bend your left leg at the knee and slowly raise your left foot up until you can grasp it with your left hand. You are now in the position of Fig. 136.

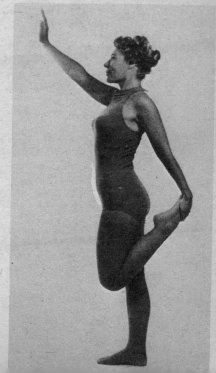

*Figure 136*

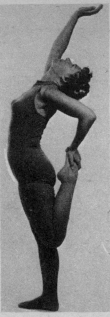

*Figure 137*

5. Now, in slow motion, perform the following movements.

   a. Pull your left foot up with your left hand.

   b. Bend your body backward at the waist.

   c. Move your right arm back as far as you can without upsetting your balance.

   d. Let your head drop slowly and gently back until you are looking upward.

6. Hold the position motionless for 10 seconds (Fig. 137).

7. To come out of *The Arm and Leg Stretch,* slowly bring your right arm forward while at the same time you release your pull on your left leg. Relieve the backward bend of your spine.

8. When you are once more in the position shown in Fig. 136, release your left foot and allow your left leg to descend to a normal standing position and lower your right arm back down to your side.

9. Repeat the same exercise on the alternate side. That is, raise your left arm into the air above your head and bend your right leg so that you grasp your right foot with your right hand, etc.

### Benefits to you

1. Your sense of balance is developed.

196

2. Improved balance results in an increase of general bodily grace and poise.

3. *The Arm and Leg Stretch* provides a delightful backward stretch of the spine, particularly in the lower part of the spine.

4. Tension in the back and thighs is relieved.

### Practice schedule

Hold the posture for 10 seconds during the first week.

Add 5 seconds each week to your holding time until you are holding it for 30 seconds.

Repeat the exercise three times on each side, alternating from your left leg to your right.

### Special hints

Remember to keep your eyes open throughout the exercise. If you close your eyes, especially when bending back, you risk losing your balance.

Possibly, in the beginning, you may lose your balance and have to either wobble to keep it or actually release your foot to catch yourself. As always, the correct thing is not to react. Neither giggle nor become irritated. Do not break the mood of serene calm that you should maintain when performing any Yoga technique. Simply go back into the posture quickly and quietly and continue as if nothing happened. In a very short while you will have perfect balance in this relaxing stretch.

# CHAPTER TWENTY-SEVEN

# Increasing Beauty and Health Through Proper Blood Circulation

## The Circulation Problem

The subject of the circulatory problem of modern people has been dealt with in some detail in *The Shoulder Stand*. In regard to circulation there is considerable similarity between the effects of *The Head Stand* and *The Shoulder Stand*. While *The Shoulder Stand* has a stronger effect upon the thyroid gland and thus upon the weight problem, *The Head Stand* has a more direct effect upon the head and brain.

The problem of improper circulation hinges on the lack of correct natural use of the body. The enormous number of people whose occupations are sedentary or insufficiently active are most liable to suffer from the results of poor circulation. The heart struggles to pump the blood against the force of gravity through the long blood vessels of the legs and back up to the heart. It struggles hard to push the blood upward against gravity through the millions of capillaries that permeate all the organs, glands and tissues of the head and brain. The portion of our bodies above the heart nearly always receive insufficient circulation. This is a chronic condition. Only active youths or athletes are immune to the problem. As soon as people slip into the rut of adult life and its unfortunate physical inactivity the condition sets in.

The results of poor circulation are devastating. They include chronic fatigue, sluggishness, lack of endurance, the feeling that the legs are heavy, no pep, no enjoyment, poor complexion, and numerous minor aches and pains. Even more than this, poor circulation brings with it the danger of major physical breakdown due to the deterioration of the circulation starved areas of the body. Poor circulation is also extremely dangerous for the heart and it has much to do with bringing about a hardening of the arteries.

The results of improved or correct circulation are as wonderfully positive as the ones I have just listed are negative. They consist of vitality, new endurance, a healthful complexion and the feeling of buoyancy, radiance and life.

*The Shoulder Stand,* which you have learned, is a superlative Yoga technique for improving and normalizing blood circulation throughout your entire body. *The Head Stand* is equally efficient but is stronger than *The Shoulder Stand* in regard to increasing the circulation to the head and brain because of the position of the neck. In *The Shoulder Stand,* the bending of the neck and the holding of the chin against the jugular notch alters the flow of blood so that it enters the head with more moderate force. In *The Head Stand,* however, the blood pours directly into the head and thus we have a more intense increase of circulation there.

## Exercise 34: THE HEAD STAND

STIMULATES AND REFRESHES THE BRAIN AND IS HIGHLY BENEFICIAL FOR THE ENTIRE NERVOUS SYSTEM. IMPROVES TOTAL CIRCULATION.

### How to practice this exercise

1. Sit in the *Japanese Sitting Position* which you have learned. (See Fig. 5.)

2. Bend forward and place your elbows and forearms on the floor. Clasp the fingers of both hands together. Do not keep your elbows too far apart but bring them in somewhat toward each other.

3. Place the top of your head on the floor so that the back of your head is snugly against the palms of your clasped hands as in Fig. 138. (See Fig. 139 for a closeup of the head and hands position.)

4. Now straighten your legs at the knees. You will then be in the position indicated in Fig. 140.

5. Walk slowly forward a few inches at a time until your knees are resting against or as close to your chest as you can bring them and only the tips of your toes are touching the floor (Fig. 141).

6. Here is one of the crucial points in the correct practice of this technique. You must push off very gently with your toes so that your feet

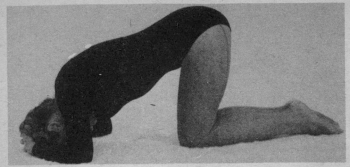

Figure 138

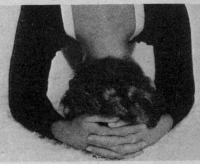

Figure 139

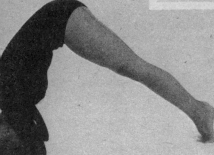

Figure 140

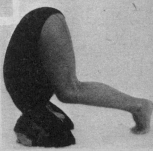

Figure 141

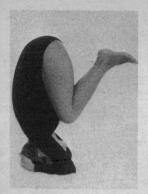

Figure 142

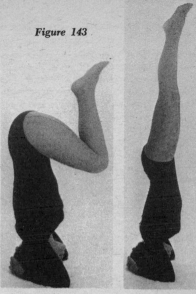

Figure 143

Figure 144

will leave the ground and your weight will be supported by your head, elbows and forearms. The mistake most people make is to kick off or push themselves up forcefully. The correct technique is simply a shifting of the last of the weight that is upon your toes over toward the triangular base formed by your hands and forearms. That is why you must inch forward as closely as you can toward your chest. Then the smallest push will enable your feet to rise effortlessly off the floor. Your thighs are still close against your chest (Fig. 142).

7. This is the position that you will hold according to the time prescribed in the practice schedule. Initially you must obtain complete control of standing on your head with your legs in this modified position or in the position indicated in Fig. 143 before straightening up into the complete *Head Stand*.

8. When you have adhered to the time requirement indicated in the practice schedule, you will next straighten your legs up into the complete *Head Stand* in which your body will be held in a straight vertical line (Fig. 144).

Slow motion is of the uppermost importance when you straighten your body up. The slower you move while straightening your legs up into the air, the surer your balance.

Hold the complete position for the prescribed time.

9. To come down out of *The Head Stand,* slowly bend your body at the knees and at the hips and in very slow motion bring your legs back down so that your knees come to rest against or as closely as possible to your chest as in Fig. 142.

10. Now lower your legs slowly and gently so that your toes come in contact with the floor without the slightest jolt. You must never allow yourself to collapse out of the posture even from the last few inches.

11. Rest on your knees and with your head still tucked between your hands for at least a minute and a half before rising.

### Benefits to you

1. Most of the benefits of *The Head Stand* and *The Shoulder Stand* are the same except that *The Head Stand* has less effect on the thyroid gland and more effect on the brain.

2. *The Head Stand* refreshes the brain by increasing circulation to all the tissues of that organ.

3. All the nerve centers of the brain are stimulated and revitalized by this flow of blood.

4. The improved circulation of blood through the brain benefits the entire nervous system.

5. The pineal and pituitary glands are nourished.

6. There is an immediate increase in your vitality.

7. The increased flow of blood through the eyes and ears is very healthy for them.

8. *The Head Stand* induces a glowing healthful complexion due to the intensified circulation through all the tissues of the face.

9. The skin of the scalp and consequently the hair roots are nourished by the improved circulation.

### Practice schedule

Hold the first position of *The Head Stand* as shown in Fig. 142 for 20 seconds during the first week.

Add 20 seconds to your holding time during the second week. Add 20 more seconds to your holding time during your third week. Thus in three weeks you will be holding the first position for 60 seconds. Do not attempt to straighten your legs up into the complete *Head Stand* until you have built up your time in the modified position to 60 seconds.

At this point you will start to straighten your body up into the complete *Head Stand.*

Begin by holding the complete *Head Stand* for 60 seconds. (That is during the fourth week.)

Add 30 seconds each week until you are holding *The Head Stand* for 3 minutes which is quite sufficient for general health purposes.

If you particularly favor this technique, you may increase your holding time to as much as 10 minutes providing that you do so at the above recommended rate of speed and no faster.

### Special hints

You should place a small pillow or several folded bath towels under your head when you perform *The Head Stand* or it might be uncomfortable for you on the hard surface. *The Head Stand* should be practiced on a moderately soft surface such as a thick rug or carpet and you would do well to spread some pillows or cushions around to soften your landing in case you tumble out of it in the beginning.

I strongly advise that you practice *The Head Stand* near a wall for at least the first few weeks. That is, when you place your head in your hands make sure the wall is about six inches or so from the back of your head. Therefore, if you lose your balance and fall toward the rear, you will simply come to lean against the wall with your feet. This will give you a sense of security in the beginning.

I caution people who are very much overweight not to practice *The Head Stand* at all until their weight has been somewhat normalized by the rest of their practice of Yoga. It is not advisable to attempt to force the neck to support excessive body weight.

Remember that the weight of your body rests on the triangle formed by your forearms, the main weight being on the elbows and forearms rather than directly on the head. Bringing your elbows a bit closer toward each other will give you better stability.

I cannot emphasize too strongly the necessity for extreme slow motion in going into and coming out of *The Head Stand*.

When you are able to perform the complete *Head Stand* for several minutes, you will experience a wonderful feeling of accomplishment.

# CHAPTER TWENTY-EIGHT

# The All-Important Art of Relaxation

## About Relaxation

The physical organism of man is very much a mimic. Like a monkey in a zoo who imitates the behavior of the people around it, the human body falls into a mimicry of the rhythm pattern of its environment. We are well aware of the difference in breathing, heart beat and general metabolism of the human body while we listen to different kinds of music. When a Bach cello sonata is being played, the heart beat and the metabolism of the body is slowed and calmed. Yet if we turn off that piece of music and turned on Count Basie and his jazz orchestra, our heart beat would, in imitation of the rhythm of the music, speed up and so would our entire metabolic rhythm. Our emotional state and mind content would similarly change. Our organisms imitate their entire environment, wherever they might be, in the same manner. That is why city dwellers go to the country where the peace alone calms the mind and body and they feel healed and regenerated. People in most modern countries live in urban environments. For countless millions of individuals it is an environment that could not be more conducive for producing jangled nerves if it had been designed specifically for that purpose. People in a city live in a basically jarring nerve-shattering world as well as one filled with the unavoidable visual ugliness of most modern cities. It is very much like living inside a great machine and our poor organisms helplessly mimic its clashing rhythm.

## The Toll of Tension

The result of living within this great machine is tension, a keyed up agitated nervous system, the forgetting of how to relax and eventually the inability to relax even when consciously trying to do so. As stated before tension and agitation produce extremely bad effects upon health and appearance.

We cannot stop the machine of the city in which we live, but we can and must stop our organisms from reacting in imitation of our environment's nerve-racking elements. Your organism must be allowed to rest in order to regenerate itself every day, but few people know how to truly rest and relax.

## Imperfect Methods of Relaxation

Everyone tries to relax but the methods usually used are imperfect and do not do the job. Some of these methods seem to provide relief, but the relief is superficial and only gives us the false impression that we are relaxed. Deep within our organism nothing has been accomplished and the cycle of tension and fatigue continues day after day.

Certain activities which would seem to be relaxing, such as shuffleboard, gardening, picnics and spectator sports, are delightful, advisable and necessary as good wholesome recreation. They remove, however, only a fraction of the tension accumulated within us. When people come home from work they often "flop" down in a chair and after a while feel that they have become somewhat relaxed. Nothing could be farther from the truth! The merest surface relief has occurred, and for a very short duration. The quick nap is another method that is indispensable to many people. It is a splendid habit but it, too, is highly over-rated when considered in the light of true relaxation. As we have indicated previously, you can go to sleep carrying all your tensions with you and wake up with the same tensions functioning in your body and mind. Innumerable people believe that sitting in a chair and watching television is good relaxation. The degree of genuine relaxation that is attained here is so minute as to be absurd. Drinking alcohol, while it may provide a quick and much needed unwinding, is equally deceptive.

## Relaxation, Beauty and Energy

Relaxation shows itself as obviously as tension does. Just as the outward signs of a tense person are negative; the characteristics of a relaxed person are positive. Relaxation shows in the face. The eyes have a warm gentle look. The features are soft. One's walk is easy and graceful and there is something about a relaxed bearing that has a soothing effect on other people.

Of uppermost importance in regard to healthful and full living is the relationship of relaxation to energy. It is axiomatic throughout the study of Yoga that tension drains a person's energy. Wherever your body is tense, that is where your vital energy is being dissipated and wasted. A relaxed body tends to conserve, store and use correctly (through the mysterious and miraculous intelligence of the human organism) the vital energy that is available to it.

## How to Relearn to Relax in Depth

Thus it is imperative for us to relearn the lost art of relaxation. You have been doing just that by learning the Yoga stretching exercises. The most penetrating, effective and long lasting method of eliminating tension from the human organism is by stretching it away. In the next technique, however, we are going to employ a different method, one which at first sight will look familiar. The purpose, nevertheless, is the same—to relax your body so that it can become "recharged" with vital energy.

You are going to learn here how to lie down and become relaxed in the limp manner. This is one of the most delightful techniques to practice and it is one that you should certainly do at the conclusion of every Yoga practice period and at any other time of the day or evening in which you feel the need for quick relaxation.

## Exercise 35: THE RECHARGING TECHNIQUE

COMMANDING EVERY PORTION OF YOUR BODY
TO BECOME LIMP. REPLENISHING YOUR NAT-
URAL ENERGY.

### How to practice this exercise

1. Lie on your back with your legs slightly apart and your arms at your sides, your hands about a foot or so from your body, palms up.

2. Keeping your body as limp as you can, perform the following movements.

Raise your left leg a few inches into the air and then allow it to fall back down upon the mat as limp as a rag. It will land with a slight bump and a bounce and you will feel an increased limpness and drainage of tension throughout that limb for that instant. Then perform the same movement with your right leg, lifting it a few inches into the air and allowing it to "flop" back onto your mat.

Bend your left arm at the elbow with your upper arm still resting on the ground and allow your left forearm and hand to fall limply down upon the mat as you did with your legs. Repeat the same movement with your right forearm.

Now raise your entire left arm a few inches up and allow it to fall in the same manner. Raise your entire right arm from the shoulder and allow it to fall.

Exerting as little muscular effort as you can, lift your buttocks and pelvis off the mat a few inches and allow that entire area to fall limply back down.

Lift your abdomen and chest off the mat, arching your back slightly, and allow that area to fall limply back down.

After going through the procedure once, repeat it a second time. At the end you should be reclining motionless with your eyes closed, as at the beginning (Fig. 145).

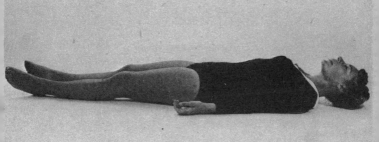

*Figure 145*

3. You will now begin to induce "deep" limpness throughout your entire body. When you finish the technique the first time you will realize the difference between becoming limp in this manner and the everyday "lying down to relax" with which you are familiar.

Concentrate your mind on your toes by thinking about them and attempting to feel them, without moving them, as in isolation from the rest of your body. Keep your eyes closed throughout the entire technique and do not move at all except as specifically instructed. Now tell your toes to become completely limp and more utterly relaxed than they have ever been before. You actually mentally order your toes to relax. Wait a few seconds and then concentrate your mind on your feet up to your ankles, thinking about your feet and no other part of your body. Command your feet to go completely and deeply limp. After a while (perhaps even from the very beginning) you will begin to feel a slight tingling in the areas which you command to relax. Wait a few seconds and let your mind rise up your legs until it includes your ankles. Command your ankles to go completely limp.

Continue to let your mind rise slowly up your body commanding each part to become completely limp and relaxed, giving each area a few seconds to do so and then moving on. Do this to your legs from the knees down. Then raise your mind up your body to your hips and command your entire legs to become inert and relaxed. Next give the order to your pelvic and buttocks region, your abdomen, your back, your chest, your fingers, your hands, your arms from the elbows down, both arms entirely, and your shoulders.

4. Your entire body below your neck is now in a state of profoundly limp relaxation.

5. Now perform the following movements in as slow and relaxed a manner as you can. Your face is looking upward. Allow your teeth to part and your mouth to open slightly. Slowly roll your head to the right until it is resting on the right side as far as it can go. Take 15 seconds to perform this movement of your head.

Now roll your head slowly all the way from where it is facing your right side to where it will be facing your left side. Take 30 seconds to perform a slow roll. Roll your head slowly back to your right taking 30 seconds to do so. Remember that your body is completely limp. Roll your head finally back until it is facing your left side again. Take 30 seconds to do this. Now tell your neck to become completely limp.

5. Lie in this position without moving and concentrate on every feature of your face and every part of your head and scalp telling each part to become as limp as the rest of your body.

6. Lie for a minimum of 3 minutes, breathing long, calm, slow breaths using your abdomen.

## About Practicing the Recharging Technique

It is an excellent practice to perform this technique as the conclusion of your Yoga practice period.

It is also a splendid technique to do during the day when you feel the need for it especially in the late afternoon or early evening. Many people practice it immediately upon coming home from work with splendid results.

# PART FOUR

# Beauty

# and Health

# Through Peace

# of Mind

# CHAPTER TWENTY-NINE

# Beauty and Health
# Through Peace of Mind

## Peace Is an Innate Condition of Man

The basic idea of Yoga regarding what we in the West have come to call peace of mind, is that peace of mind and spirit is the natural state of man. Thus it is not something we *add* to ourselves. Peace is a state of being that is realized. It is like clearing away weeds on land that is already your own and finding underneath a treasure that was always there. The peace for which all people universally yearn is an innate condition in every human being. All human beings who experience true peace realize, at that moment, that it was always within them, only waiting to be discovered. It is an error to search for it outside of one's self.

## What Is Peace?

Peace is a condition of human completion to which certain qualities or characteristics can be attributed. One of these qualities is equanimity, or the ability to treat good and bad fortune with the same attitude and with emotional calm. The person with equanimity is not crushed by events or blasted with disappointment.

## What Characterizes the Absence of Peace

The symptoms of what we can call lack of inner peace are as commonplace as the ground we walk on. They include anxiety, worry, fear, hate, guilt, habitual irritation, temper, strife and a kind of pathological discontent. These symptoms, when listed in this manner, turn out to be quite a dismal picture. Yet, most people carry any number of these characteristics within themselves every day of their life. A person doesn't think of attempting to eradicate them directly until they reach a degree of intensity that is unendurable. I assure you that the "normal" amount of these symptoms which the average person possesses is quite sufficient to erode the very foundations of his life and to make happiness and peace of mind seem to ever-recede before him.

This way of thinking is natural while under the pressure of these inevitable problems of living, and the idea that the changing of the outward conditions around us will in itself cure them is a fundamental fallacy.

The root cause of all these problems is known to Yoga and it lies *within* the individual, inside you. It is there that you must go in order to find the basic cause of all the problems of life.

The inward journey is a great adventure which results in the one shining achievement of humanity—true and lasting peace of mind and spirit.

## The Lost Horizon of Serenity

One cannot attain peace of mind simply by developing the correct traits or presumed characteristics. That is as much a facsimile of peace as simply sitting cross-legged in a Yogic position and staring straight forward is in itself only the merest facsimile of Meditation. The true and real peace of mind which the Yogi speaks is not a going forward and attaining something new and never before possessed by the individual. It is a *return* to a condition that is already there by nature, which has always been there, but which has been forgotten and come to be covered with a number of obstructing characteristics.

Thus the science of Yoga occupies itself with the removal of obstructions that obscure the perfect attributes that already exist rather than the adding of characteristics to the individual. Peace of mind, liberation from the wheel of life, Nirvana, awakening, enlightenment, the experience of Universal Mind (call it what you will, every name given to this state of being means the same thing) is experienced by the individual in the form of a remembrance. It is somewhat analogous to the unique experience of turning a corner in a city in which you have never been before and recognizing the street and every house and every stone just as if you had lived there at some time. In the case of the experience of true peace the recognition takes place because you have been there before. You have always been there. Liberation from the wheel of life and peace of mind is the natural state of man. Indeed you are there now. You could not possibly ever be anywhere else. You simply are not aware of it. Your ability to directly experience true peace is covered by the notion of being a separated ego-entity and subsequently you are subject to all that that unfortunate notion brings with it.

All you have to do regarding the experiencing of peace of mind is to practice the mental techniques of Yoga in order to realize your basic nature.

## Mental Exercises (Raja Yoga)

*The Way Is Meditation.* Meditation is a synonym for the term Raja Yoga. It is the universal form of mind control being the common denominator of all known systems and variations of mind control.

Meditation means control of the mind substance, a concept virtually unknown in the West. With all the volumes that have been written on psychology by the greatest psychologists and psychiatrists in the Western world, I have yet to come across an authoritative comment on the subject of mind substance. Yet the subject of mind substance has been known and investigated completely in the East for thousands of years.

The idea of mind substance is simply that the mind is composed of something. Obviously the mind is an extremely ordered and systematized mechanism. It will act consistently all the time. Even insanity is a consistent and ordered reaction. Now if there exists an entity which is ordered and which functions and reacts in an ordered and systematized manner, then it has to have a structure. That is, it has to be made of parts which function together like the systems of the physical body and which adhere to very specific and exact mechanical laws.

The substance of which the mind is made is refined indeed. In the West we would perhaps call it electro-magnetic force, but it is obviously there and is as real as the solids, liquids and gas of which the physical body is made. One of the primary characteristics of the mind substance is movement. It is always moving. The task of mind control is not to manipulate the subject matter—the thoughts or concepts—of the mind. The object of mind control is to quiet the primal restlessness of the very substance of which the mind is made.

In India a pool of water is used as a symbol of the mind. When the water in the pool is moving or agitated, then one can only see the ripples, or movement itself, of the water. One cannot see into the body of water nor through it to the bottom. One can only perceive a very limited aspect of the nature of the water. If the water is allowed to settle—to set so that its movements become slower and eventually stop completely as the water settles into a diamond-like stillness—one can see *into* the body of the water and *through* it. This is representative of the everyday mind. So long as the substance of the mind is uncontrollably moving, you cannot see into its essential nature. When, however, one enables the substance of the mind to slow down, to become calm and eventually to be still, then one sees into the essence of the mind and one sees through and beyond the mechanical mental apparatus, transcending it and its limitations.

The first step to the attainment of this basic quietude of mind is called concentration. Concentration is the ability to place all of the conscious attention upon one point to the exclusion of any extraneous mental activity. The only reason that this is considered difficult is because we in the West are never taught the correct natural way of achieving concentration. Actually it is extremely simple.

## How to Stop Thinking

The way to mind control is to develop the ability to temporarily stop thinking. Many a person in the West is amazed when they first hear that a Yogi can stop thinking for a number of minutes or longer. There are usually many who look upon it as a feat of enormous difficulty, which again is not the case at all. It is as simple and mechanical as learning to play the piano. Learning it depends upon methodical regular practice. The absence of thought does not bring about a state of voidness. It is not a lack of total awareness, but simply the stopping of the uncontrolled flow of conceptional thinking and the endless parade of wasteful, worthless fantasy and talking to one's self, that goes on nearly every moment of the waking day. Concentration of the mind upon one point and the stopping of the wayward thought processes constitute the first necessary step on the path to true inner peace.

Therefore we will begin with an exercise that develops both of these abilities.

### Mental Exercise 1: THE CANDLE CONCENTRATION EXERCISE

#### How to practice this exercise

1. This exercise must be performed in a completely dark room. Sit on the floor in a cross-legged position. Place a candle so that the flame is at eye level and at approximately one arm's distance directly in front of you. The only light in the room should be the light of that candle flame.

2. Gaze at the flame for three minutes. You can approximate the time and you will invariably come within seconds of it. Blink normally

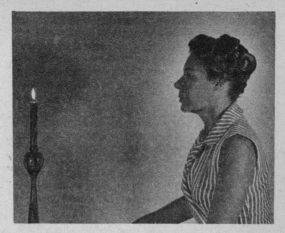

*Figure 146*

but do not look away from the candle flame. Attempt all the while to prevent extraneous thoughts from entering and occupying your mind. If a thought begins to arise in your mind and distracts your concentration simply bring your attention back to the flame in a relaxed manner (Fig. 146).

3. When you have done this for at least three minutes, take your hands and cup them over your eyes so that no light whatever can reach your eyes. Do not close your eyes but keep them open and stare into the total darkness of your cupped hands.

4. You will then see the after-image of the candle flame before you.

The object of the exercise is to keep the after-image visible for as long as you possibly can. It usually lasts no longer than three minutes. The after-image of the candle flame will tend to drift out of your vision and sometimes to fade and become smaller and more distant. When it does, simply compel it to reappear by making an additional effort at concentrating. It will reappear for a number of times before finally fading entirely away. While performing this concentration upon the after-image, you should continue your attempts to prevent any thoughts whatever from occupying your mind.

Besides developing the ability to concentrate the mind on one point and to clear the mind of extraneous thoughts, this technique is extremely soothing to the nervous system. You will find it immensely relaxing and able to "unwind" you after a tense day.

## Mental Exercise 2: MEDITATION ON THE BREATH

The candle concentration exercise is an excellent preparatory technique for Meditation. *Meditation on the Breath* is an ancient Raja Yoga technique that has been practiced for centuries by countless persons for the very same reason for which we use it today.

The breath plays an uppermost part in mind control because the breath itself has a direct control over the mind. When the breath is quick, short and wavering, the mind cannot be at rest. On the other hand when the breath is slow, smooth, and quiet the mind automatically tends to slow down and to become quieted, calm and serene.

That is why I strongly urge you to perform the *Alternate Nostril Breathing* exercise previously described immediately before practicing this meditation technique. Indeed, to obtain the utmost results from your meditation you should make *Alternate Nostril Breathing* part of your meditation by performing at least seven rounds of *Alternate Nostril Breathing* and then, at the conclusion of your last round, go directly into your meditation.

*Meditation on the Breath* calms the metabolism, the nervous system, and the emotions. It quiets the mind, clearing it of all thoughts of anxiety and worry that come to prey upon it during the day. The ability to concentrate is developed and you achieve a control that results in serenity of mind and joyful quietude of spirit.

### How to practice this exercise

1. The first step in *Meditation on the Breath* or in any form of passive meditation (that is meditation which is performed sitting alone in a quiet private place) is to sit cross-legged and erectly.

2. The second step is to perform seven rounds of *Alternate Nostril Breathing* using *The Complete Breath* throughout.

3. The correct use of the eyes is essential in meditation. The eyelids must be lowered but not closed. You should be able to see only the circle of space in which you are sitting.

Next you must focus your eyes inward until you are looking at the tip of your nose. This may be uncomfortable in the beginning for some people due to the fact that they are not used to crossing their eyes. The idea that crossing the eyes is bad for you or dangerous is a myth. Actually once the eye muscles become accustomed to the position, it is quite relaxing. If you feel a slight discomfort at first, then do not focus your eyes all the way in to the tip of your nose but focus them outward eight or ten inches. Then in a day or two when your eye muscles start to become accustomed to the position, you can slowly feel your way in toward a complete inward focusing. Inward focusing of the eyes has a two-fold purpose.

First you draw attention away from the objective world. This in itself is a relief from the continuous demands upon you. It thus becomes a gateway to entering into one's self. Its second purpose has to do with helping the student concentrate his mind upon the one point that is called for in this technique, the breath.

4. Sitting correctly in a cross-legged position with the breath having been slowed, deepened and steadied and the nerves calmed by *Alternate Nostril Breathing*, practice *Meditation Upon the Breath.*

Breathe long slow quiet breaths and as you do so perform the following:

## (a) OBSERVE YOUR BREATH

Concentrate your attention upon the place from which the air is drawn into your nostrils from the atmosphere around you. Attempt to visualize the current being sucked slowly and gently into your nostrils. In the beginning you can follow the course of air as it proceeds down into your lungs, fills your lungs and then is slowly exhaled. During your exhalation keep your attention upon the place at which you visualize the breath emerging from your nostrils and merging once again into the ocean of air around you. When you are able to do this without your mind being carried away by extraneous thoughts, you can concentrate your attention solely upon that place where the air enters and leaves your nostrils.

## (b) DO NOT ALLOW ANY THOUGHTS AT ALL TO ENTER YOUR MIND OR IN ANY WAY DISTRACT YOUR CONCENTRATION ON YOUR BREATH

You'll find in the beginning that your mind will trick you. You will discover suddenly that in the midst of your Meditation you are really not sitting there in the room and enjoying the great relief on your mind and nervous system but you are back, for example, on Main Street again reliving some incident. Your mind has taken you somewhere else other than the place of Meditation. When this happens, the rule is—do not react. React no more than you sensibly should if you were learning to play the piano and your finger struck a wrong note. You don't waste time with an emotional reaction or with scolding yourself. When a slip occurs, forget it immediately and come back to where you were before you made the mistake. Do not recognize the fact that your mind has tricked you and distracted you during Meditation. Simply focus your attention back upon your breath and continue as if nothing happened. You will find in a very short time, usually within two to three weeks of daily practice, that the tendency of your everyday mind to wander off and occupy itself with its usual trivialities will grow less and less and very shortly you will be able to meditate undistractedly.

### (c) COUNT YOUR BREATHS

After every nine breaths begin counting over again at one in order to prevent time from lagging unnaturally due to our lack of habitual practice in sitting silently and still. It also prevents the student from becoming drowsy during meditation.

Never close your eyes during meditation. If you do it will tend to make you sleepy. Meditation is actually the process of bringing about a higher awakening, not a sleepy or trancelike state.

Meditation is really as simple as it seems. Once again, however, we see how complexity itself has very little relationship to profundity. The highest truth and the most profound activities are characterized by simplicity.

## Controlling Random Thoughts

Thoughts will continually attempt to push their way back into your attention during Meditation. This will happen more frequently in the beginning of course but you will gain great control over tendency as you practice. Remember that only one thought can exist upon the stage of your attention at one time. Here is man's greatest advantage in the challenge of mind control. It means that you are not obliged to deal with a multitude of thoughts pouring through your mind at the same time. As a few weeks go by and distracting thoughts come to occupy your attention less and less during Meditation, you will experience a feeling of both relief and triumph. You know that you are no longer helplessly subject to the tyrannical imposition of fruitless thoughts and fantasies; you are no longer a leaf blown helplessly before every habitual self-indulgent wind of your mind.

You will then see that this incredible and natural form of self-mastery has opened the door to peace of mind and spirit.

From all the many students to whom I have taught physical and mental Yoga I have invariably been told of two results of Meditation. The first is that the students very quickly come to experience a new and wonderful kind of peace and tranquility. They are no longer susceptible to aggravation, nervousness or severe emotional reaction in the face of life's complications. They tell me how they have come to be calm in the midst of confusion. The second thing that they inform me of is—and this is usually with a gleam of enthusiasm in their eyes—that some person who has known them for years has come up and asked them what has happened. When they inquire what they mean, their own friend invariably says, "Why you seem so different, so calm, and so relaxed."

Of all the students to whom I have taught Meditation I have never heard any report other than this. After a few months of practice, your physical demeanor as well as the air about you will be one of beautiful serenity.

# PART FIVE

# Practice Schedules

# and Special Programs

# CHAPTER THIRTY

# A General Schedule That Can Be Used as a Lifetime Exercise Program

*Morning Schedule*

1. The Cleansing Breath (always done in combination with The Complete Breath) in The Half-Lotus position.
2. The Abdominal Contraction.

You can perform half your Abdominal Contractions in the same sitting position in which you perform The Cleansing Breath. Then perform the second half of your Abdominal Contractions in the standing position.

3. The Arm and Leg Stretch.
4. The Cow.
5. The Standing Twist.
6. The Side Bends.
7. The Chest Expansion Posture.
8. The Backward Bend.
9. The Backward Bend On the Toes.
10. The Knee and Thigh Stretch.

This morning schedule is designed to work out the kinks that have come to lodge in your body during your night's sleep, limber your body, wake and alert your mind and senses and energize you. You will be amazed and gratified at the effectiveness of the morning routine. It sets you up for the entire day, sending you into your day's work feeling fresh and alive.

## Afternoon Schedule

1. Cleansing Breath (as always with its accompanying Complete Breath).
2. The Cobra.
3. The Neck Stretches.
4. The Locust.

Remember that you will be starting with the Half Locust as instructed in the exercise, before you shift over into practicing The Full Locust.

5. The Bow.
6. The Ankle to Forehead Stretch.
7. The Forehead to Heels Stretch.
8. The Spread Leg Stretch.
9. The Alternate Leg Pull.

You should not perform the Variation of the Alternate Leg Pull until you are able to go completely into the Alternate Leg Pull where your forehead rests on your knee and your elbows rest on the floor beside your extended leg. The Variation of the Alternate Leg Pull is an advanced technique and is only meant to be practiced when you have gained sufficient flexibility.

10. The Leg and Back Stretch.
11. The Plough.
12. The Twist.
13. The Lion.
14. The Shoulder Stand.

You will practice the Head Stand here in place of the Shoulder Stand according to your preference or if you happen to be adhering to one of the *Practice Schedules for Special Problems.*

15. The Eye Movements are optional depending upon your particular need for them.
16. Alternate Nostril Breathing.

If you do the Alternate Nostril Breathing at night before retiring, then you may eliminate it from your afternoon schedule if you are pressed for time.

17. The Recharging Technique.

You must adjust your afternoon schedule to your time limitation. If your time is short, feel free to do only two repetitions of the exercises that are less important to you and which do not apply as significantly as others to your major health and beauty problems.

Figure 147

*HILDEGARDE, the internationally famous singer, beginning the PLOUGH. HILDEGARDE not only practices Yoga regularly but is a noted authority and an author on the subject of health.*

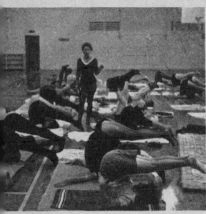

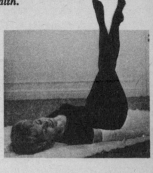

*igure 148*

*ve Diskin instructing one of her classes in e practice of the PLOUGH.*

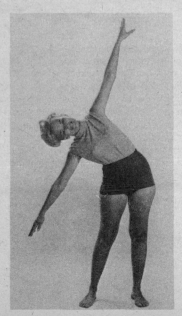

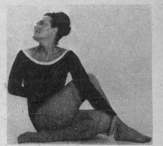

*Figure 149*

*Figure 150*

*Yoga Programs for Special Problems*

## A YOGA PROGRAM FOR THE WEIGHT PROBLEM

These special programs only apply to your afternoon exercise period. You should keep your morning schedule the same all the time.

1. The Abdominal Contraction.
2. The Cleansing Breath.
3. The Shoulder Stand.
4. The Cobra.
5. The Plough.
6. The Twist.
7. The Side Bends.
8. The Cow.

If the weight problem is your main health and appearance concern, you should begin every daily exercise period with the techniques listed here. Place your greatest emphasis on these eight exercises and practice them with your fullest enthusiasm and with devoted regularity. After you have practiced these particular exercises, go right on with the rest of your regular afternoon schedule, only do not repeat these particular exercises where they would normally have come.

If time is of the essence, you should practice these eight techniques completely and slowly but you can adjust the rest of your techniques to your personal schedule, for example, repeating a number of the others only two times instead of three.

The Shoulder Stand is of uppermost importance in application to your weight problem. You should build your time of holding The Shoulder Stand up to five minutes. This combination is extremely effective for coping with excess weight. You will hamper its effectiveness, however, if you do not make a sensible adjustment in your diet. I recommend eliminating white sugar and all white sugar products from your diet. You should also eliminate white flour and all white flour products, including commercially made cakes and candy of any kind. You should go easy on bread and potatoes especially in combination with meats. You should eliminate animal fats from your diet and substitute vegetable oils in their place. Stop eating desserts. Substitute honey and molasses for the sugar. This alteration of your diet, when applied specifically in combination with the Yoga exercise program, should begin to show wonderful results in a very short time.

## A YOGA PROGRAM FOR THE TENSION PROBLEM

1. Alternate Nostril Breathing.

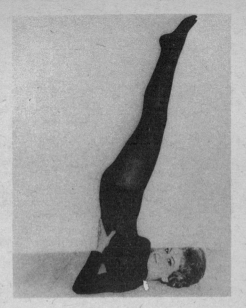

*Fig. 150A*
*OLIVIA DE HAVILLAND executing the SHOUL-*
*DER STAND.*

Perform it in whatever Yoga sitting position is most comfortable for you.

2. The Cobra.
3. The Neck Stretches.
4. The Lion.
5. The Forehead to Heel Stretch.
6. The Alternate Leg Pull.
7. The Leg and Back Stretch.
8. The Shoulder Stand.
9. The Eye Movements.
10. The Recharging Posture.

The instructions regarding the starting of your regular daily Yoga exercise period with these techniques apply to all of the special problem practice schedules. Begin your afternoon workout with the exercises that are recommended for your special problem. Apply yourself most diligently to them and then complete your workout with the rest of your daily techniques.

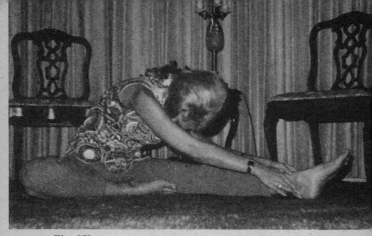

*Fig. 151*
*A housewife stretching herself free from tension with*
*the ALTERNATE LEG PULL.*

## A YOGA PROGRAM FOR THE STIFFNESS PROBLEM

1. The Backward Bend.
Perform the backward bend until you are flexible and comfortable
in it. Then work your way from The Backward Bend into The Backward
Bend on the Toes.
2. The Cobra.
3. The Chest Expansion Posture.
4. The Alternate Leg Pull.
5. The Spread Leg Stretch.
6. The Plough.
7. The Leg and Back Stretch.
8. The Twist.

## A YOGA PROGRAM FOR THE FATIGUE PROBLEM

1. The Head Stand.
If a reason such as age, fragility, or infirmity prevents you from performing The Head Stand, you should substitute The Shoulder Stand in its
place.
2. The Chest Expansion Posture.
3. The Cow.
4. The Cleansing Breath in combination with The Complete Breath.
5. The Locust.

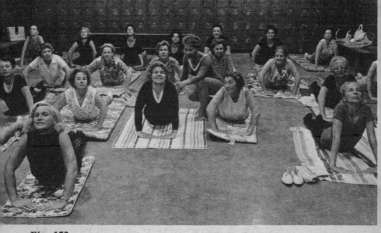

Fig. 152
A class learning how to free their bodies from tension
with the COBRA posture.

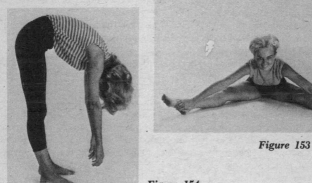

Figure 153

Figure 154

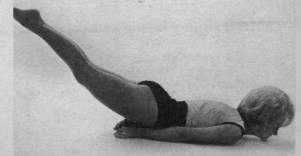

Figure 155

## A YOGA PROGRAM FOR A TIRED FACE

1. The Shoulder Stand.
2. The Plough.
You can go directly into The Plough from The Shoulder Stand.
3. The Lion.
The Lion posture is of uppermost importance for the face. You should perform at least the required three repetitions but you may feel free to increase the number of repetitions of The Lion according to how much need you feel for it. You cannot overdo this particular exercise.
4. The Neck Stretches.
5. The Cow.
6. The Eye Movements.

## A YOGA PROGRAM FOR BETTER SLEEP

1. The Shoulder Stand.
Do not perform The Shoulder Stand within one hour of going to bed for the night. It is best performed from one to two hours before retiring.
2. The Neck Stretches.
Special emphasis should be placed here on The Slow Neck Drop and on warming the eyes (with the use of a light bulb).
3. The Eye Movements.
4. The Candle Concentration Technique.
This technique is optional.
5. Alternate Nostril Breathing.
You should perform this exercise when you have already turned out the lights and lain down to sleep for the night.
A superlative practice to help improve sleep is for you to drink a glass of hot herb tea with one or two tablespoons of honey in it before beginning these final nighttime techniques. Delicious herb teas are easily available.

## A YOGA PROGRAM FOR IMPROVING YOUR POSTURE AND BEARING

1. The Backward Bend.
2. The Cobra.
3. The Backward Hand Clasp.
4. The Standing Twist.
5. The Arm and Leg Stretch.
6. The Chest Expansion Posture.

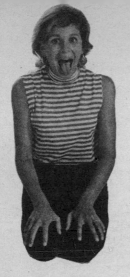

Figure 156

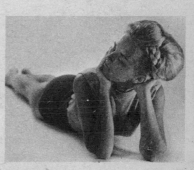

Figure 157

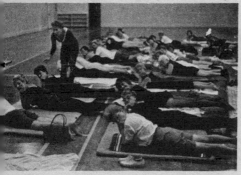

Fig. 158
Students experiencing the wonderful relaxation that only Yoga gives.

Fig. 159
As part of your program to improve your sleep, do the SHOULDER STAND one hour before retiring.

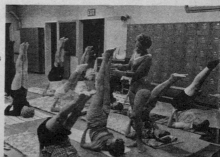

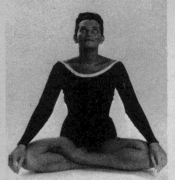

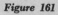

Figure 161

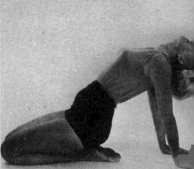

Figure 160

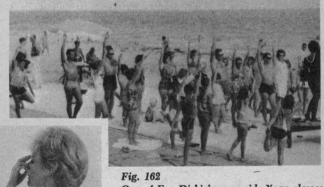

Fig. 162
One of Eve Diskin's oceanside Yoga classes
doing the ARM AND LEG STRETCH. A
perfect combination for lifelong youth and
fitness; Yoga, sunshine and fresh sea air.

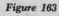

Figure 163

## A YOGA PROGRAM TO OVERCOME
## THE CIGARETTE HABIT

1. The Cleansing Breath in combination with The Complete Breath.

Perform this first thing in the morning and also as the first and the concluding exercise at every Yoga exercise session. If possible you should practice this combination of techniques just before every cigarette you smoke. While it is somewhat difficult to do, if you can make yourself remember to do one or more sets of Cleansing Breath-Complete Breath combinations every time that you reach for a cigarette, the results will be simply amazing.

2. Alternate Nostril Breathing.

Perform this every night when the lights are out and you have lain down in bed to sleep.

## A YOGA PROGRAM FOR THE NERVES

1. Alternate Nostril Breathing.

Perform the exercise after every Yoga workout. Do it every night upon retiring. Besides this specific technique the best thing you can do for your nerves is to practice a full schedule of Yoga stretching exercises every day.

2. Meditation on the Breath.

Meditation is a superlative antidote for frayed nerves.

# Epilogue

If an ounce of prevention is worth a pound of cure, then a few minutes of Yoga each day is indeed worth the risk of physical debilitation and breakdown that attends neglect of proper body care. The idea of prevention has always been associated with Yoga. Patanjali, one of the supreme Yoga sages, said in the second century B.C.,

*"The trouble that has not yet arrived, that is what is to be avoided."*

We would like to compliment you on the beauty and health-consciousness which has led you to the study of Yoga. This beauty and health-consciousness represents a high degree of wisdom and farsightedness. If you practice regularly as you have been instructed, you will inevitably reap the wonderful benefits that are yours at the minimum expense of effort and time.

Sincerely,

*Eugene S. Rawls and Eve Diskin*

# Index

## A

Abdomen, beauty and health for the, 88-96
  about the abdomen, 88-89
  plough exercise for, 89-94
Abdominal Contraction Exercise, 189-193 (*see also* Regularity)
  benefits of, 191
  how to practice, 189-191
  practice schedule, 191-192
  proper peristaltic action in colon, 189
  technique for natural regularity, 13
Age, and the practice of yoga, 23-26
  helps in sports, 23-24
  older people and need, 24-25
  school, children and students, 23
  yoga always working for, 25-26
Air of Life About Oneself, vitality, and feminine beauty, 4
Alertness, interest, and beauty, 4
Alternate Leg Pull, 58-62
  benefits of, 56
  practice schedule of, 56
    fig. #16 to #20, 58-60
  special hints, 56-57
Alternate Nostril Breathing, and nerves, 180-186
  benefits of, 182-183
  calming body and mind, 180
  entity of body and mind, 184-185
  how to practice, 180-182
    fig. #129-131, 181-182
  old ideas of breath control and emotion, 185
  practice schedule, 183-184
  scientific breath control and emotions, 185-186
  special hints, 184
Ankle to Forehead Stretch, 80-82
  benefits of, 82

Ankle to Forehead Stretch (*Cont.*)
  how to practice technique, 80
  fig. #33-35, 81-82
  practice schedule, 82
  special hints, 82
  stretching hip area, 80
Arm and Leg Stretch Exercise, for balance, poise, 195-197
  arms, flabby and shapeless, 4
  benefits of exercise, 196-197
  how to practice, 195-196
    fig. #136-137, 195-196
  practice schedule, 197
  special hints, 197

## B

Back, beauty and health for the, 111-118
  about the back, 111
  bow exercise, 115-118
  complete leg and back stretch, 112-114
    benefits of, 114-115
    practice schedule, 115
    special hints on, 115
Backward Bend, for the feet and ankles, 43-46
Backward Bend of the Toes, 33-38 (*see also* Toes)
Backward Hand Clasp, 121-122
  benefits of, for the back, 121
  how to practice, 121
    fig. #78-79, 122
  practice schedule for, 121-122
  special hints, 122
Balance, increasing (*see* Poise and Grace)
Bearing, stiff, inflexible, 4 (*see also* Poise and Grace)
Beauty
  aims of yoga for, 1

233

# EVERY YOGA FAN WILL WANT TO READ . . .

**YOGA FOR YOUR LEISURE YEARS** (82-152, $2.25)
by Eve Diskin

**A HANDBOOK OF YOGA FOR MODERN LIVING** (89-596, $1.95)
by Eugene S. Rawls

**BE YOUNG WITH YOGA** (89-432, $1.95)
by Richard Hittleman

**JOY OF LIFE THROUGH YOGA** (76-736, $1.25)
by Eugene Rawls & Eve Diskin

**RENEW YOUR LIFE THROUGH YOGA** (89-515, $1.95)
by Indra Devi

**YOGA FOR BEAUTY AND HEALTH** (82-972, $2.25)
by Eugene Rawls & Eve Diskin

**YOGA FOR PERSONAL LIVING** (89-433, $1.95)
by Richard L. Hittleman

**YOGA FOR PHYSICAL FITNESS** (89-099, $1.95)
by Richard Hittleman

---

**W** A Warner Communications Company

------------------------------------------------------------

Please send me the books I have checked.

Enclose check or money order only, no cash please. Plus 50¢ per copy to cover postage and handling. N.Y. State residents add applicable sales tax.

Please allow 2 weeks for delivery.

WARNER BOOKS
P.O. Box 690
New York, N.Y. 10019

Name ..............................................

Address ...........................................

City ................. State .......... Zip ..........

_____ Please send me your free mail order catalog